SOMATOEMOTIONAL RELEASE AND BEYOND

JOHN E. UPLEDGER
D.O., O.M.M.

ILLUSTRATIONS BY
FRANK LOWEN

PALM BEACH GARDENS
UI PUBLISHING, INC.

2003

First Printing 1990
Second Printing 1994
Third Printing 1995
Fouth Printing 1996
Fifth Printing 1999
Sixth Printing 2003

DEDICATION

To all of you who have been trusting and kind enough to allow me to blend with you and grow.

John E. Upledger
D.O., O.M.M.

Table of Contents

FOREWORD

SomatoEmotional Release and Beyond is a landmark book. The author presents a leading edge exploration of mind-body relationships, using the idiom of touch. He describes the actual process of his journey into previously undefined territories of the human body. Through this journey he brings to us an alternative methodology for investigating the world of health and disease.

In his book, Dr. Upledger shares his own evolving understanding of the whole person in a manner that opens new possibilities for the patient/client, the therapist/facilitator and the medical community. The author takes us beyond the boundaries of his own scientific and medical training, allowing his personal experience to become his guide and ours for further learning.

As he explores body-mind relationships through touch, he uses both his imagination and communication skills to define his experiences and share them. He presents new concepts, a new vocabulary and an expanded view of the human body-mind. As Dr. Upledger defines "unwinding," "energy cyst," or "SomatoEmotional Release," new words and new concepts for most of us, the information becomes immediately accessible and applicable. Each new concept becomes a stepping stone for still another discovery, with author and reader seeming to share in the excitement that comes with such disclosures.

SomatoEmotional Release and Beyond is invaluable as are the author's insights. They help validate many nontraditional realities and experiences that bodyworkers frequently encounter: the impossibility of separating mind from body, the reality of an "energy" within the body, the interrelationships of our own thoughts and feelings with the experiences of the client.

In the Western world of science and technology, we are taught to look outside ourselves for knowledge and verification. We are implicitly or explicitly encouraged to distrust personal experience. Scientific investigations that follow Koch's postulates for setting up and verifying information in a laboratory setting, for example, still hold a supreme position in the medical community.

In light of recent discoveries and observations in science, however, especially in the science of advanced physics, we have begun to accept the fact that these so-called "objective" methods of observation may not be as dependable as we once thought. We now know that the subtlest thoughts and intentions of researchers have an effect on the outcome of the experiment. We cannot truly separate the observer from the observed. In medicine, we know that thoughts and intentions dramatically affect a person's inner environment, the immune system, for example. Ultimately, we have come to understand that we simply cannot objectify others nor the dynamics that affect their health.

Dr. Upledger uses a different methodology than Koch's postulates for identifying cause; his methodology offers us more complete access to the whole person. He uses his own experience as the investigating probe and the responses of his patients/clients—both their subjective reports on each process and their body responses—as his feedback loops. The author keeps readers informed of his processes, formative discoveries, doubts and the evolution of his thinking. Throughout, he guides us, sharing his journey as he probes deeper and deeper to reveal the unknown.

How this book is received will depend upon the reader's personal experience. At times the author risks invoking disbelief because he moves so fast and is so very candid. He presses our imagination to look beyond more traditional paths of investigation. Yet when we consider his credentials, his background and his stories, it is difficult to dismiss his observations even if they are outside our own experience.

At this point in history, it has become evident that the issues of health extend beyond the limits and responsibilities of the allopathic medical profession. It is necessary that others with alternative ideas to help meet the challenge of world health step into the arena. After reading this book, it is clear to me that Dr. Upledger is one of these people. His book deepens our understanding of the whole person and opens new pathways to improved personal health.

Fritz Smith, M.D.
Watsonville, California

After reading John Upledger's newest book, *SomatoEmotional Release and Beyond,* I reread some of A.T. Still's comments on fascia. Dr. Still states in his 1899 *Philosophy of Osteopathy:* "I know of no part of the body that equals fascia as a hunting ground. I believe that more rich golden thought will appear to the mind's eye as a study of fascia is pursued than any division of the body."

Many osteopathic physicians have read this statement by the founder of osteopathy in the U.S.A. but few have taken the time to allow intuitive perceptions about fascia to be followed by active research on the subject. Few have used the outcomes of their research to develop clinical teaching models for students. Even fewer have spent their time and energy to write three books on the subject as John Upledger has with CranioSacral Therapy.

This third volume updates John's growing relationship with fascia as an integral partner to help create and maintain wellness. In this book he demonstrates the importance of fascia as a part of the storehouse for tissue memory of all kinds. He also has shown that fascial-related tissue memory can become a messenger to both the client and the facilitator for deeper insight and understanding of the self-healing process.

It appears that the cells of our bodies possess holographic information that can be transmitted from our untapped inner resources (nonconscious state) to our conscious state of awareness. The hands-on interaction of the client and facilitator in a SomatoEmotional Release session provides one of the most complete body-mind-spirit opportunities for this to take place. The Energy Cyst model has, by research and empiricism, been the foundation for this conceptualized idea.

You will enjoy the contents of this book because it possesses the harmony of practical hands-on instruction from the factual brain; i.e., additional techniques for manipulation of the hard palate, tongue and submandibular tissues in balance with the perceptual information and multiple case study experiences in the realm of the Energy Cyst, SomatoEmotional Release and Vectoring.

The associations that John makes with his knowledge of Chinese pulse diagnosis, acupuncture meridians and related organs, as well as with Kirlian photography, allow the facilitator to access other stores of knowledge he may have to assist the hands-on healing process.

John has learned much about imaging and dialogue from teachers such as Martin L. Rossman, M.D., in his book *Healing Yourself*. The broad spectrum of examples in imaging and dialogue in John's book will help push back our walls and make room for greater freedom in our client-facilitator interaction. This will allow those with whom you work to be as elaborate or simplistic as they choose in visualization.

The Significance Detector has given major enhancement to the client and facilitator relationship because it establishes a confidence factor within the facilitator and, therefore, their interaction together. John's discussion of the facilitator's role in the client process toward wellness is an imperative for all practitioners of SomatoEmotional Release. The goal of physical-mental-emotional-spiritual cooperation is demonstrated in this book with the result of a unified awareness toward wellness for all. Dr. Still states: "We can see all the beauties of life on exhibition by that great power with which fascia is endowed. The soul of man with all the streams of pure living water seems to dwell in the fascia of his body."

You will find John Upledger's most recent endeavor an adventure—a search for truth. I think that you will also find that it can help further your own personal and professional growth.

Richard C. MacDonald, D.O.
Palm Beach Gardens, Florida

INTRODUCTION

The pressure to write a book on SomatoEmotional Release[sm] has been present and increasing since 1985. Finally in December of 1988 I could no longer procrastinate and the process began while we were in Hawaii. If you are going to describe a process that is progressing at a dizzying pace, you just have to start somewhere. I did, and you'll see why as you complete your perusal of this book.

As is my wont, I have begun with a description of the history and development of the concepts and techniques of SomatoEmotional Release as they are laid out before me. Then I have attempted to describe the concepts of Energy Cysts and SomatoEmotional Release as they are today. Of course, today is now yesterday—and tomorrow will be today in the very near future. When you undertake the description of a dynamic process that seems endless, whatever you write about it on whatever day you write it will be yesterday's news by the time the text goes to press, so please understand the futility of attempting to achieve an up-to-date description of events which are the subject of this book.

It felt very necessary to document a how-to-do-it description of the Vector/Axis system. This has been done. Some of the people who have read this chapter have said they now understand vectoring, whereas they did not understand the workshop explanations. I have even included some sample problems in this chapter so that left brain types can take heart.

The chapter on Therapeutic Imagery and Dialogue is long, but I think it is chock full of helpful ideas and suggestions for bodyworkers who, as they work, discover that the body and mind are inseparable and actually just different facets of a single, unified being. If you get into the body a little deeper than the very superficial symptomatic treatment, you will discover the mind. I have tried to describe what you can do as you encounter the patient/client's mind to help the therapeutic process to continue and keep you out of trouble. There is and will continue to be great controversy about the boundaries within which a therapist can work, depending upon his/her credentials. In my opinion, this controversy cannot be resolved until there is a general recognition that if the mind and body are not a single entity, they are—at the very least—so integrated and intertwined that no amount of legislation or rule making can cause them to be separate entities, with one in the domain of the "mindworkers" and the other in the domain of the "bodyworkers." As the bureaucracy struggles with this artificial separation, patients/clients continue to suffer. Trust the process; help people; subordinate your ego and stay out of jail.

Subsequent to all of this, I felt that I owed it to you to let you see some of what has happened to me in my lifetime that has taken me to where I am today. Hence the chapter titled "Personal Growth Experiences." These are events, experiences and observations which have helped me to open my mind. It is not my intention to convert or evangelize. It is my hope that my sharing perhaps will give you food for thought. I began my osteopathic medicine career rather focused, tunnel visioned and perhaps myopic. The lessons that were set out before me required only that I gain some modicum of patience so that I could observe without interference and hysterical rationalization. All I needed to know was that I didn't know and wouldn't/won't know until the time is right.

Finally, we get to the "beyond" of *SomatoEmotional Release and Beyond*. The chapter titled "Some Call It Channeling" recounts, as accurately as I can recall, some of my experiences with patients. It is presented for you to make of it what you will. These things happened. How you choose to explain them is your choice.

I do hope you enjoy this book. I suggest you read it in its entirely first, then go back and study its parts. Enjoy!

The next book is already entering my consciousness.

Best personal regards to all of you.

John E. Upledger, D.O., O.M.M.

Chapter I
SomatoEmotional Release:
The Evolution of a Concept

DEFINITION

SomatoEmotional Release (S.E.R.) is the expression of emotion that, for reasons deemed appropriate by some part of the patient's or client's nonconscious,[1] has been retained, suppressed and isolated within the soma. We might think of the soma as the "somatic psyche." Observation of the S.E.R. process suggests that independent retention of the energy or memory of both physical and emotional trauma is frequently accomplished by specific body parts, regions and viscera.

We initiate the S.E.R. process by hands-on communication between therapeutic facilitator and patient/client. It is the result of meaningful and intentioned touch. The meaning and intention of the touch may be either conscious or nonconscious.

Psychiatrists and psychotherapists who have witnessed or participated in the S.E.R. process often liken it to body psychotherapy. In this analogy we see the patient/client's body movements as analogous to the verbal aspect of psychotherapy. From clinical observation, it would appear that most somatically retained trauma and emotion originally occurred against a background dominated by physiologically destructive emotion such as anger, fear or guilt. This destructive emotional background may have been either acute or chronic.

Personal observation of and participation in hundreds of S.E.R. processes has led me to postulate that organs, tissues and perhaps individual cells possess memory, emotional capacity and intellect. Release of retained tissue emotion and pain usually passes through the patient/client's conscious awareness either at the time of the S.E.R. experience or within 24 to 48 hours. Conscious recall of past incidents connected to "isolated" tissue memories most frequently occurs as sudden insight within a few hours if not at the time of S.E.R.. It is not uncommon for patients/clients to consciously experience tissue-related emotion at the time of S.E.R. and to have recall of the original incident later.

---

[1] The word "nonconscious" is used throughout this text to denote any somatic, mental or spiritual process or situation not within the patient's conscious awareness at the time described. The word was coined to avoid the wide variety of connotations—correct or incorrect—which have accumulated around the words "unconscious" and "subconscious."

DEVELOPMENT OF THE S.E.R. CONCEPT

SomatoEmotional Release is not something that was intellectually conceived. The idea developed as the result of multiple experiences in different places that all began to point toward the same central focus. In the late 1970s, I was a principal investigator in research at a county center for autism. We aimed our work at the question of the possible efficacy of the use of CranioSacral Therapy in the treatment of autism. At the same time I was working with Zvi Karni, a biophysicist and bioengineer on loan to our department at Michigan State University from the Technion Institute at Haifa, Israel. Dr. Karni and I were investigating and successfully measuring the effects of my therapeutically intended touch and manipulative procedures upon the baseline electrical potential of the human body. Concurrently, I was seeing several private patients/clients outside these research settings.

AUTISTIC RESEARCH

The first year of our work with autistic children focused on observations of their characteristic behaviors and personalities, as well as physical examinations and craniosacral and structural evaluations. We also conducted blood, urine and hair analyses. There were 26 children in our research project. We studied the children's responses to our attempts to move into their private worlds—that are, at least on the surface, very isolated and personal.

We observed that gentle, non-intrusive, well-intentioned touch was the most acceptable entry. We also discovered that "Still Point"[2] induction by the use of this accepted gentle touch helped to establish a positive rapport between the autistic child and ourselves. Our team was made up of myself, Dianne L. Upledger and Jon D. Vredevoogd as well as an ever-changing stream of interested and dedicated graduate students. Some of these students were from the Osteopathic College at Michigan State University and some were from related healthcare colleges. We all did hands-on work and began to appreciate and know the value and potential of well-intentioned touch.

During the second year of this research project, we began exploring various therapeutic approaches. We used nutritional counseling with parents and guardians. We modified the physical environment in terms of lighting, temperature and humidity. We used 10 percent CO_2, 90 percent O_2 inhalation therapy to stimulate deeper breathing. We used a variety of indicated manual therapies for structural mobilization and corrections. Last but not least, we applied CranioSacral Therapy once a week to each child.

Over the years, it has become clear to me that I can learn much more by observing than I can by invading. This was not always true of my approach. During my first 10 years in private general practice and emergency room coverage, I was an invader *par excellence*. "Make it happen," was my motto. Fortunately, I tempered that attitude to some extent, and I became 90 percent observer and 10 percent invader in our craniosacral work with autistic children. The progression of events with most autistic children in our research project went something like this:

---

[2] "Still Point" in this context is a therapeutic interruption of craniosacral rhythm which allows the craniosacral system to reorganize its activity for more optimal effect on the body. The Still Point may be imposed from outside by a therapist or may be a spontaneous homeostatic process. It may occur very suddenly by a precise alignment of the body in a significant position or by the experience of a significant emotion. In this way, it can function as a "Significance Detector": John E. Upledger, *CranioSacral Therapy II, Beyond the Dura* (Palm Beach Gardens: UI Publishing, 1987), Chapter IV: Section 2d. The Still Point helps balance the symmetry of the craniosacral system and corrects many restrictions in this system in a nonspecific way; it reduces sympathetic tonus, enhances fluid exchange between physiological compartments, reduces stress, lowers fevers and enhances the body defense mechanisms against pathogens. It is an efficacious, wide spectrum natural therapeutic event.

First, the establishment of rapport and trust was imperative. We did this patiently and quietly, first by touch and then by the induction of Still Points wherever our hands were touching the child. We frequently induced Still Points at the knees, the shoulders, the feet or the arms. We could seldom use the head for the first several sessions. Our first few sessions often took place on the floor under the treatment table. It was wherever the child wanted to be, wherever he or she would allow us to touch his or her body. Sometimes, the autistic child would allow only one of us at a time to touch him or her but almost without exception, three or four of us eventually were able to touch the child at the same time.

Not infrequently, these autistic children would object violently to the touch of one of us but allow touch from another. This response made us aware of the power of the intention of the "toucher" and how it is nonconsciously or consciously broadcast to the "touchee." I could, on occasion, sense negativity in a graduate student. When I did become aware of any negativity, I excluded that student from touching until a positive attitude was generated. Occasionally I had to exclude an assistant with a negative attitude from the treatment room. The autistic children clearly demonstrated the ability to discern the therapeutic facilitator's intent and attitude. I'm sure that on some level they also understood the effect that attitude and intent might have upon their being.

Conversations with research physicist Neil Mohon suggest that we all have multiple and qualitatively different energy fields that belong to each of us individually. Mohon's research over the past 15 years has been in the area of energy field detection devices. He believes that each human being may have as many as 50 different personal energy fields. Since energies may either attract or repel, he suggests that the most successful therapists/facilitators have energy fields that are attractive to a greater proportion of people. That is, the successful therapeutic facilitator's energy field has the least repellent potential. Sensitive organisms such as pet beagles will automatically be attracted to or withdraw from certain individuals. This may be due to the nature of the projected energy. Autistic children may possess the same sensitivity. I believe, and Mohon agrees, that once the therapeutic facilitator is aware of his/her energy field potential they can modify it by intention or thought projection.

After the successful induction of Still Points on several visits, the autistic children usually became cooperative and of their own volition would assume a supine position upon the treatment table. Then I would proceed to work with the child's head very gently and tenderly. Because focus is so important, I always concentrated on loving that child at that time. Slowly, I would add my assistants to the therapeutic session by having each one hold an individual upper or lower limb. Ultimately, five of us usually treated a single, allowing and cooperating autistic child during each CranioSacral Therapy session. Most sessions lasted for 20 minutes. Today, I feel that longer and more frequent craniosacral sessions would have produced much more dramatic results, but we were working under rather inflexible time constraints.

As we treated each child, it seemed that after a few preliminary cranial vault releases, we always encountered a severe membranous anterior-posterior restriction of the floor of the cranial vault. This was decompressed by first lifting the frontal bone and maintaining the lift until we could sense the viscoelastic[3] change that signified the membranous release between the frontal and sphenoid bones. Next, we decompressed the sphenoid from the occiput. It was during this procedure that I began to more fully appreciate the restrictive potential of the sutural articulations between the petrous parts of the temporal bones and the sphenoid anteriorly and the occiput posteriorly. The sphenobasilar synchondrosis was but a small part of the restriction of the floor of the cranial vault. There was a lot of osseous and membranous release to obtain before the floor of the vault became functionally mobile. Yet in most cases the floor of the cranial vault was successfully anterior-posterior decompressed.

Almost immediately in these decompressed children there occurred a great reduction or total cessation of self-abusive and self-destructive behavior. By this, I mean that the children voluntarily stopped banging their heads against the wall or they stopped biting their wrists or hands or they stopped gouging that favorite part of their body. It was as though the reason for self-inflicting pain activity no longer existed.

One can develop several viable hypotheses for this dramatic behavioral change. The most attractive hypothesis to me is that the compressed and restricted cranial bases of such children cause a deep, out-of-control pain inside their heads. Head banging and thumb pressure on the roof of the mouth—which was often mistakenly interpreted as thumb sucking—could be instinctive attempts to release the cranial base restrictions. Chewing on the wrist and otherwise gouging the flesh were, perhaps, attempts at either inducing elevated endorphin production, closing the Melzack-Wall pain gate or substituting a controllable pain for an uncontrollable pain. Perhaps a combination of these possibilities was in effect.

After—and only after—the successful anterior-posterior decompression of the floor of the cranial vault and the reduction or total cessation of self-abusive behavior did the next most remarkable and instructive phenomenon occur: After the release of the anterior posterior compression, it became apparent that there was severe medial compression of the temporal bones bilaterally. It was through our

---

[3]   Viscoelastic property of tissue refers to that characteristic response of connective tissue which may be described as initially elastic and later viscous when a load is applied: John E. Upledger and Jon D. Vredevoogd, *CranioSacral Therapy* (Palm Beach Gardens: UI Publishing, 1983), pp. 128 – 30.

attempt to decompress the temporal bones by moving them laterally that two very useful happenings occurred. First, we devised the "Ear Pull"[4] technique for temporal decompression. Second, and most significant to the origin of the concept of SomatoEmotional Release, the child's body began to move autonomously—that is, an arm or leg would show a tendency to move as though it had a mind of its own. We decided to follow these movements rather than try to inhibit them. (Remember, I was usually working with four assistants, one on each arm and one on each leg.) During the times that these spontaneous body movements were occurring, lateral decompression of the temporal bones seemed impossible. This was why I began to pull gently on the ears. It made good sense to me because the ear is attached to the temporal bone via its connective tissue continuity between the pinna and the ear canal. This connection went from the outside to the deeper parts of the petrous temporal bone where the internal end of the canal opens to admit the facial and vestibulo-auditory (7th and 8th) cranial nerves.

I was unsuccessful in decompressing the temporal bones laterally, but as we continued to work and gently try for temporal decompression, the amount of patient/client-induced limb and body movement continued to increase. This was not conscious, voluntary movement. It seemed automatic. By this stage of the treatment process the autistic child was typically in a deep state of relaxation and the body was very loose and relaxed except for the subtle movement tendencies just described. These subtle movements occurred only when one of us held the involved body part. They usually began with a limb and then slowly they would spread to involve the torso, the neck and the head. We followed and we became extremely sensitive to intended body movement. Without our following and lending physical support, the movement would stop. It was as though the therapeutic facilitator's touch imparted the necessary energy to initiate the body movement process. The continuation of the process depended heavily upon our ability to follow the most subtle body intentions, counteracting the forces of gravity without leading or inhibiting the child's body movement. As our skills developed, these autistic children's body movements went further and further until they would reach a position that seemed an apparent end point, a place where everything became quiet and still. This end position could be either anatomically normal or quite abnormal.

I remember a child's right foot pointing directly posterior. It was rotated about 180 degrees at its end point. He went into this position of his own volition and stated when questioned that he was very comfortable with it. (Later, after the

---

[4] The Ear Pull Technique refers to that method of mobilization of the temporal bones which makes use of gentle posterior-lateral traction applied to the pinna of the external ear. See pp. 127 – 128 and 180 – 182 of *CranioSacral Therapy* for a full description of this technique.

CranioSacral Therapy session, he could not achieve this anatomical position and would not allow us to put him into it.) As we waited at this point—and we did wait because we didn't know what else to do—there came a palpable release throughout the body. It was as though his body had opened. As muscles softened, fascia and connective tissues lengthened and fluids and energies began to flow more freely, the child cried. It was at these end points, while we were waiting, that total body release would occur. The child in question might cry softly or wail very loudly. We saw what looked like expressions of fear, anger and frustration coming out of these children. These expressions, both facial and postural, often continued for several minutes as body releases processed. When the releasing process was nearing completion, the facial expression typically became more peaceful and loving. Once initiated, these events seemed to occur more than once on each of several visits with each child. In each subsequent session the releases seemed less intense until finally no more "spontaneous" body motions occurred. Then and only then could I successfully decompress the temporal bones laterally. I still cannot give a plausible explanation for the relationship between medial temporal restriction and the release of body tension and emotion that we observed.

Inability to express love and hold affection for other humans is a hallmark of autism. After the releases of both body tension and emotional expression, these autistic children typically began to express affection toward other human beings. Another hallmark of autism is withdrawal from social contact. These children would demonstrate sociable behavior and begin to play with classmates.

We didn't know it at the time, but we had witnessed and participated in our introduction to SomatoEmotional Release.

BIOELECTRICAL MEASUREMENTS

While the autistic research project was under way, I worked independently with Dr. Zvi Karni in an attempt to measure electrical potential changes in the patient/client's body that might correlate to various therapeutic activities. We investigated the effects of acupuncture, various types of osteopathic manipulation and CranioSacral Therapy (as it was later named) on these electrical potentials.

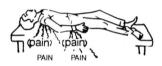

A. Patient in pain

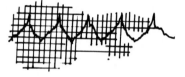

Electrical potential during pain

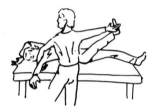

B. Patient/client's body moves into therapeutic position. Craniosacral rhythm stops. Therapist/facilitator holds the therapeutic position until craniosacral rhythm begins again.

C. Craniosacral rhythm begins. Body is allowed to move to any position it indicates. Processes in "B" are repeated as necessary.

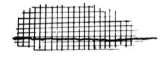

Electrical potential while craniosacral rhythm is "shut down."

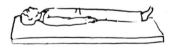

D. Pain is gone. Body returns to "normal" position.

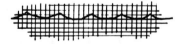

Craniosacral rhythm is in motion. Electrical potential activity is soft and regular.

Correlations between body positions, electrical phenomena and subjective pain relief.
Illustration I – 1

We had begun our joint project as adversaries. I had challenged any one of our engineers and biophysicists to try to measure what I subjectively had perceived as a transference of some type of energy from therapeutic facilitator to patient/client or vice versa during the treatment process where the therapeutic facilitator rested the hands on the patient/client (bare skin not required) for 30 seconds or more and without performing any gross movement. At the time I put this challenge to the departmental faculty members, I had only a few months seniority as a research clinician in a Department of Biomechanics made up of five clinicians and 22 Ph.D. researchers from a variety of disciplines. The charge to the department was to use interdisciplinary means to investigate the previously unexplained observations made by the clinicians during their years of practice. We had weekly Wednesday morning meetings chaired each week by an expert in experimental design. The disciplines represented by the Ph.D. group ranged from anatomy to psychology to biophysics. It was in this setting that I suggested we try to measure an exchange of energy between patient/client and therapeutic facilitator during a hands-on treatment session. At first I was politely refused; later not so politely refused. I persisted in the presentation of this possible focus for research and was ultimately a source of laughter. I didn't take kindly to laughing and became adamant, suggesting that perhaps the problem was too difficult for these physicists and engineers to tackle.

This approach got a response from Dr. Karni who allowed that he would work with me long enough to prove that, at least on this question, I was a crazy imbecile with delusions of grandeur. We began.

First Dr. Karni simply came in as an observer while I was seeing clinic patients. Since I was viewed as a specialist in biomechanics, most of my clinic patients were people suffering from long-standing pain. We normally thought that this pain was neuromusculoskeletal in origin and most often related, according to the referring doctors, to some sort of injury or trauma. Dr. Karni called to my attention that a large portion of my treatment consisted of placing a patient's body or body part in a position that created a reduction or total ablation of the patient's subjective sensation of pain. I usually held the patient in this position until certain cues indicated to me that the positive effect was complete. Then I would reposition the patient's body on the treatment table and go about further evaluation to determine whether any direct technique would be carried out to mobilize an immobilized, "stuck" joint. More often than not, after repositioning the patient nothing further was necessary. I had, apparently on an intuitive level, developed my own system of "position and hold"[5] technique.

---

[5] Later, I became acquainted with the work of Larry Jones, D.O., who also came upon the concept of "position and hold." His work evolved into Strain/Counterstrain. One of his early articles is published in *CranioSacral Therapy*, Appendix E, pp. 300 – 310.

After several hours of observation and rather agonizing question and answer sessions between Dr. Karni and me (it is difficult to realize how little you can explain of what you are doing), we decided to consider the measurement of electrical potential inside the body. Inherent in this approach was the model of the body as a skin-enclosed bag of electrically conductive fluids and tissues. (Later we would view the fascia as a specialized micro-conduction system within the skin.) In this model the skin is acting as an insulator between what is inside and outside it. We conveniently considered the skin acupuncture points as valves that would permit the flow of electrical energy to pass in or out in a homeostatically controlled manner. On occasion these valves needed adjustment, using needles or other methods of external stimulation. We did not hypothesize that the purpose of acupuncture points was necessarily to conduct electrical energy through the skin, but it did and still does seem reasonable that this is the function of some of these points. Anyhow, we viewed the skin as the insulator barrier that maintained the differential in electrical potential between the constituents of the body it enclosed and the external environment.

After some trial and error, we found that when we algebraically added the electrical "noise" that electromyographers routinely tune out, organized patterns of predictable change during the usual sequence of treatment events were displayed. Dr. Karni achieved this algebraic addition of electrical potential deviations by manufacturing his own instrument that he inserted between the patient and our multichannel recording machine. Dr. Karni's device was fashioned after the classic Wheatstone bridge with which most of us became familiar in the undergraduate physics laboratory. The noise of electrical activity was high until we reached the body position that offered subjective pain relief to the patient. At this point in the treatment process, the electrical noise abruptly diminished and the baseline of electric activity moved toward zero on the tracing. It remained smooth and near zero as the "tissue release" progressed.

As it seemed appropriate to move from the "therapeutic position" (unbeknownst to me as I was positioned so I couldn't see the polygraph tracings), the baseline of the electrical potential moved a little away from the zero line and some "noise-like" electrical activity returned. Seldom was this noise as great as that which was presented before finding the therapeutic position and obtaining pain relief. Usually the degree of pain improvement was inversely correlated to the amplitude of the noise and the elevation of the baseline after the position for the relief of pain was realized.

After what seemed like a tremendous amount of work, observation, badgering, argument and discussion, I was finally forced by Dr. Karni to realize that the physiological cue upon which I was unconsciously reliant for the discovery of exactly the correct position of the patient for pain relief was the absolute and sudden cessation of palpable craniosacral rhythm. As the craniosacral rhythm subtly began to return in the patient's body, I sensed a relaxation of tissues and a release of heat as well as a sense of fluid and energy flow through the body part I held. As these subtle phenomena occurred I repositioned the body in a way that seemed comfortable and appropriate for that individual.

We observed this sequence of events on several occasions as the body position, subjective pain and changes in electrical inside-the-skin phenomena occurred in concert. We played lots of games with each other to test the interdependency of these variables. Without any cue from me, Dr. Karni would mark on the polygraph tracing when he thought I had found the right position for the therapeutic release. He set up a screen with he and his polygraph on one side, my patients and me on the other. He could not see what I was doing and I could not see him or his tracings. Dr. Karni developed the aptitude to view the tracings and tell me what I was feeling and doing with the patient. He also could accurately tell the patient when subjective pain relief occurred. And we continued. By now we were friendly. We didn't know what we had stumbled onto, but it was exciting.

We could see on a polygraph tracing, tuned to measure fractions of a millivolt, the levels of electrical potential inside the skin. (We used silver-silver chloride electrodes on the skin. We did not penetrate the skin.) We could see the changes in electrical potential that occurred when the craniosacral rhythm stopped. We could see from the electrical potential when pain relief occurred: The electrical potential could tell us how long the therapeutic facilitator should maintain the specific therapeutic position that seemed to offer pain relief.

The next big question loomed unavoidably. Why should a very specific body position offer permanent pain relief for a situation that had begun several years before that and had been symptomatically troublesome and disabling for a long time? Not far behind was the next question: Why or by what mechanism does the craniosacral rhythm abruptly stop when we obtain the therapeutic position? How and why do the observed patterns of electrical changes occur in relation to these phenomena?

We decided to work on the big question of body position and pain relief first. It was pursuit of the answer to this question that led us to a concept of "Energy Cysts" that we teach today. In all honesty, I have no satisfactory answers to explain the mechanisms by which the craniosacral rhythm stops nor the inside-the-skin electrical potential changes that occur in the therapeutic position. Many possibilities have come to mind over the years, but none really rings true. Let's consider at this time the Energy Cyst model that does ring true to me, to Dr. Zvi Karni and to Dr. Elmer Green of the Menninger Foundation. (In fact it was Dr. Green who actually suggested the name "Energy Cyst" for the process/condition as I described it some years ago to his research group at the Menninger Foundation.)

THE ENERGY CYST MODEL

As I worked with Dr. Karni observing, he forced me to realize that somehow I was helping the patient's body reach a position, contorted or otherwise, that offered pain relief. More often than not, relief was permanent. How did this come about? Observation indicated that in the correct position—and it had to be correct, to the millimeter—pain relief was accompanied by a tissue softening, a total body relaxation, a reduction of the pulmonary respiratory rate and effort, a palpable increase in fluid and energy flow through the involved body parts (by involved I mean those body parts used to achieve the correct position) and a release of heat at some rather localized area which I frequently had at least partially covered with my hand. We came to call this correct position the "therapeutic position" for obvious reasons. And when we got to the therapeutic position, the craniosacral rhythm stopped and electrical potential changes occurred. Our question was about the reasons why a given, precisely correct body position allows or induces these changes.

Dr. Karni directed me back to the work of Erwin Schrödinger, a prominent German physicist of the first half of this century who contributed generously to the concepts of today's quantum physics. Dr. Schrödinger is largely responsible for the concepts of entropy and negentropy (or information). Our discussions led us to

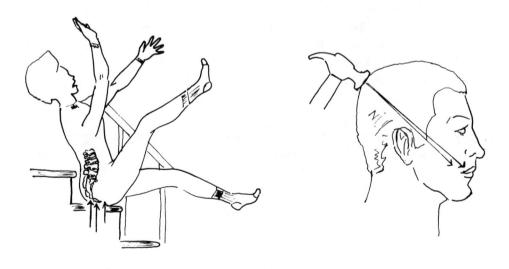

Arrows indicate direction and penetration of force vectors as they
enter the body during a traumatic experience. See text.
Illustration I – 2

the idea that a traumatic injury is, in physical terms, an injection of energy into the victim's body; for example, a blow on the sacrococcygeal complex when a fall is suddenly interrupted by a stair step. Granted, the stair step also suffers a blow from the sacrococcygeal complex but the stair step is probably the less vulnerable of the two colliding masses. The motion between the two structures at the time of collision is relative. It matters little whether the sacrococcygeal complex goes down to meet the stair step or the stair step comes up to meet that body part, the effect is the same. Another example is a blow on the head dealt by a hammer in the hands of a mugger. The head may not be in motion. All the relative movement may be provided by the mugger driving the hammer to the head.

In both of the above examples, energy is injected into the victim's body: In the first case by the stationary stair step and in the second by the moving hammer in the hand of the mugger. The quantity of energy and that energy's forward momentum as it enters the recipient's body are counterbalanced by the dampening effect of the bodily tissues the energy penetrates. This dampening effect relates to the viscosity or density of the tissues in the traumatic energy's path. If there were no dampening effect, the energy of the injury would simply go right through the victim's body and come out the other side. This is not so. Body tissues have density and, therefore, they provide a dampening effect that the momentum-driven injury force must penetrate. The distance of penetration is the result of the relationship between the quantity of force and its momentum and tissue density.

$$\frac{\text{Traumatic Force}}{\text{Tissue Density}} \quad \text{x} \quad \text{K} \quad = \quad \text{Distance of Penetration}$$

Equation which illustrates the relationship between traumatic force, tissue density and distance of penetration. K is the constant that converts this equation from qualitative to quantitative.
Illustration I-3

The energy imparted by the patient/client's collision with the stationary stair step or with the hammer will penetrate into each body a given distance. This distance of penetration is proportional to the amount of force in the blow and is dependent upon the types of tissues it must penetrate. Where the energy of the injury rests is answered by the equation in Illustration I-3. Keep in mind that for practical purposes this energy of injury penetrates the body in a straight-line trajectory. It does not go around corners. If we were to envision the duration of time of the actual collision between the stair step or the hammer and the body as about one-fifth of a second; and if we were to envision that the energy of injury entering the body, not in a continuous stream, but in quantum parcels of one one-hundredth of a second each; then, if we were to envision that the body is in motion because of the impact of the injury, we can see that we could hypothetically have 20 parcels of energy entering the body, each with its own straight-line trajectory to make up the one-fifth-second duration time during which the collision forces were operative.

If the body began its movement response to the injury force after five-one hundredths of a second and continued moving throughout the balance of the duration of the collision, this would mean that the initial five parcels of energy would share the same straight-line of energy trajectory, while each of the subsequent 15 energy parcels would have independent and slightly different trajectories. The initial delay in bodily movement response is attributed to inertia. As the body moves in response to the collision, the movement causes each previous straight-line trajectory to become bent. The next energy parcel makes its own new straight-line trajectory that is immediately bent and rendered obsolete by the body's continuing motion response. Our model requires that the trajectory path of traumatic force entry must be straight in order for the injury energy to exit the body the same way it went in. If the trajectory path of entry is bent, the injury energy is trapped at the end of its penetration.

Once this energy enters the recipient's body, it must be dealt with. It is an abnormal input of excess energy. It is disruptive to the controlled, functioning energy systems of the body. Dr. Karni and I conceptualized the human body as a skin-enclosed bag of electrical conductors with various coefficients of conduction. We envisioned the body fluids as very conductive, and we saw the connective tissues as possessing specific properties of conduction for micro-currents that somehow nurture these tissues. (We also saw acupuncture meridians as specialized lines of conductivity within the tissues.) This model begins to suggest the existence of specialized conductive qualities present in specific conductor tissues that match certain electrically energetic systems.

Anyhow, we reasoned that the energy of injury penetrated the body tissues to the appropriate depth at which location the body was confronted with the question of what to do with these 20 parcels of unwanted energy. Externally derived, this energy is disorganized and chaotic. It does not fit into the bodily organization of the intrinsic energy systems. The unwanted energy may lodge in a viscus such as the brain, the bowel or the heart. Once there, it can disrupt visceral function. Or, it may lodge in the connective tissue, bone or joints and cause pain as well as dysfunction. Wherever it lodges, it will disrupt efficient function. If it is able, the body's first choice is to dissipate this disruptive energy. The next best choice is to localize it. When localized, it creates problems in the smallest area possible. The intrinsic energy systems must then work around this localized area of disorganized energy. This accommodation of the extrinsic disorganized energy comes at some cost to the victim's total body—but the expenditure is necessary.

Dr. Karni and I thought of the localized area of extrinsic disorganized energy as an area of increased entropy as described by Erwin Schrödinger in the 1930s.[6] Dr. Schrödinger hypothesized that entropy could be—and is—reorganized by intelli-

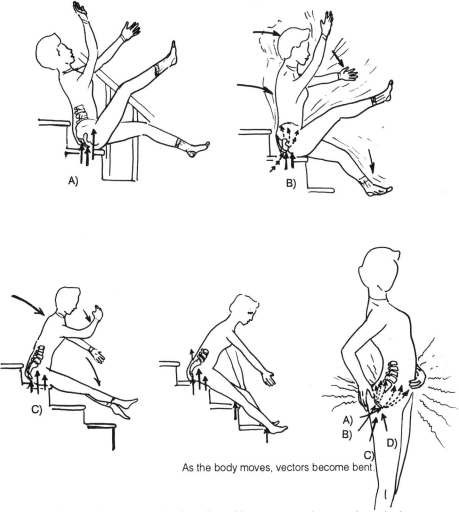

As the body moves, vectors become bent.

Arrows demonstrate the bending of force vectors (entry trajectories) as body position changes during the duration of impact with the step. This creates multiple Energy Cysts at different locations. Illustration I – 4

[6] An excellent description of Schrödinger's concepts of entrophy and negentropy can be found in his book: Erwin Schrödinger, *What is Life*, second edition (Cambridge: Cambridge University Press, 1967). The first edition was printed in 1944. In 1958 it was published again in a single volume with another of Schrödinger's works, *Mind and Matter*. If you locate this volume, please get one for me too. I'll be happy to pay you for it.

gent means in biological systems. He called this "reorganization information." In short, the unbridled progression of entropy results in total disorganization and chaos. In a biological system, this results in death and decomposition. Biological systems, however, can reverse or inhibit the progression of entropy by using "information" to cause a reorganization or release of this energy so that it can be used for the restoration of function within the system.

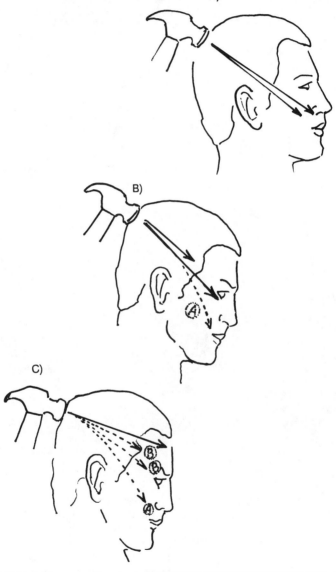

Hammer blow to the head introduces vectors as described in text.
Trajectories are bent as the head moves in response to the blow.
Illustration I – 5

Dr. Karni suggested that I was reading the patient's body signals (intelligence) and assisting in the provision of information by attaining the therapeutic position that resulted in the release of the excess, disorganized, highly entropic, disruptive energy. The release of this unwanted energy was analogous to the providing of information into a system of increased entropy. It resulted in improved function and remission of pain. (As I described this conceptual model to the research staff at the Menninger Foundation in Topeka, Kansas, Dr. Elmer Green, the research director, put his hand in the air at the back of the room. I called on him to hear his question. Dr. Green said, "John, you have just described a cyst of energy." The name stuck.)

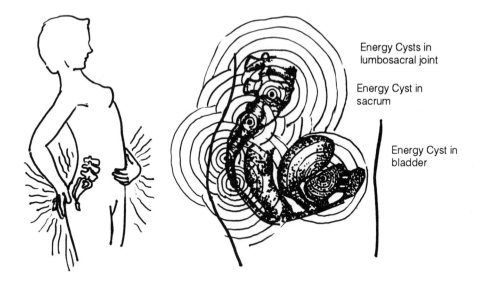

Energy Cysts in
lumbosacral joint

Energy Cyst in
sacrum

Energy Cyst in
bladder

Multiple locations of Energy Cysts. Each is released via the body position that provides a straight exit pathway for this trajectory. Thus the body position of entry must be mimicked.
Illustration I – 6a

Back to our model. It seemed reasonable that the exact positioning of the connective tissue would align the fibers so that it would enhance normal micro-current flow and allow escape of disorganized or excess energy from the Energy Cysts to the exterior surface and then out of the body. We saw and felt this phenomenon as heat during the release that occurred while in the therapeutic position. As we realigned the connective tissue fibers to improve conduction coefficients, we allowed entropy to reduce/escape.

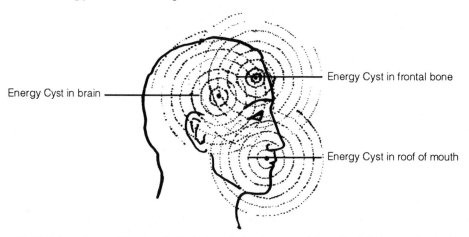

Multiple locations of Energy Cysts in head after hammer blow. Each is best released in the body position present at the time of entry. This makes the energy trajectories straight.
Illustration I – 6b

Dr. Karni used the example of the copper wire to help me understand what he felt was happening. As we know, copper is an excellent conductor of electricity. If we hit a copper wire with a hammer, we reduce its conductivity somewhat. If we can successfully and correctly stretch the copper wire to realign the particle arrangement within the wire (the blow of a hammer causes some disorganization of the particles), we can restore full conductivity to the wire.

He felt, and I agree, that it is feasible that the same phenomena can occur with connective tissue. We realign the fibers in the therapeutic position to allow improved conduction and the extrusion of unwanted foreign and external energy.

We then added to our model the idea that the most efficient escape route for each energy parcel injected during the collision was the exact trajectory of entry. So each trajectory of entry temporarily had to be reestablished to allow the release of its specific energy parcel in the reverse direction from entry—hence, the several very closely related positions of therapeutic release during a single session.

It appeared that each energy parcel had to be released along its own original entry pathway. The hypothetical stair step and hammer injuries described above each involved 20 parcels of energy. Before the body overcame inertia and began to move in response to the collision, five parcels went into the body from each impact. Then after body movement began, each parcel of the last 15 in the individual injuries had its own slightly different trajectory. Therefore, to obtain full therapeutic effect there would be 16 therapeutic body positions of release for each of the two injuries to obtain full therapeutic effect from the approach. It follows, therefore, that there would be 16 positions of the body around the sacrococcygeal complex and 16 positions of the head at which the craniosacral rhythm would stop. The electric potential baseline would drop and smooth out as all the other phenomena of release occurred. (Your job as therapeutic facilitator is to very sensitively follow the patient's body movement tendencies, discover the therapeutic positions and very patiently wait for the release phenomena to move to completion in each position.)

Another phenomena that frequently accompanies the attainment of the therapeutic position and release is the expression of emotion related to the injury. There is frequently a re-experiencing of the incident/injury or collision by the patient/client. It is as though the Energy Cyst has stored within it the memory of its creation and the emotion that was present at that time. As the patient becomes aware of the emotion and goes through the re-experiencing, the last effects of the Energy Cyst are completely dismissed. The patient now can view the whole incident in a symptom-free condition with a certain emotion-free, objective detachment.

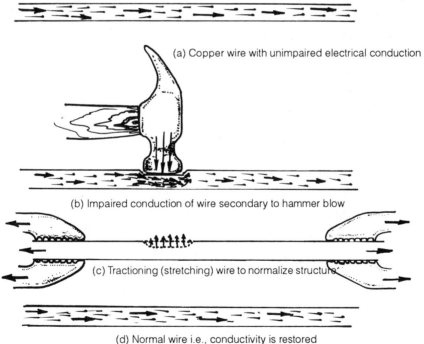

(a) Copper wire with unimpaired electrical conduction

(b) Impaired conduction of wire secondary to hammer blow

(c) Tractioning (stretching) wire to normalize structure

(d) Normal wire i.e., conductivity is restored

Effect of hammer blow (b) and tractioning (c) of copper wire
upon the wire's conductivity. See text.
Illustration I – 7

For example, the patient/client who slipped on the stairs and landed at the bottom on the sacrococcygeal complex may have experienced fear, panic and/or anger because of the slippery steps instantaneously with the realization that she/he was falling. These same feelings would be felt during the release of these Energy Cysts. In the case of the hammer blow from the mugger, similar emotions may have occurred and would be released with the Energy Cysts. This emotional release seems to be very significant to the total therapeutic effect.

Another obvious question if this model is to hold up is: What were the conditions that favored healthful dissipation of the energy of injury, and what were the conditions that favored retention of this energy as an area of increased entropy that we now call an Energy Cyst?

Clinical observation led us to the concept that a background of destructive emotions such as fear, anger or guilt favors Energy Cyst formation, whereas a background of constructive emotion—love, joy and happiness, for example—favors dissipation of the extrinsically imposed energy followed by normal healing and rehabilitation. The destructive emotional background could or could not be related to the specific injury. For example, if the person who fell off the stairs onto a concrete walkway were running out of the house in a very elated state of mind to greet a long lost friend and did not have enough fear or panic to overpower such happiness at the instant of the fall, the injury probably would heal without residual effects related to Energy Cyst formation and retention. If, on the other hand, that person were running out of the house to escape from the yelling of an irate spouse, the energy of injury would more likely penetrate and be retained as an Energy Cyst. The same would be true of our mugging victim. A person in a good mood who didn't see the hammer blow coming would suffer the immediate physical damage but probably not form a retained Energy Cyst. This does not mean there would not be significant brain damage and related dysfunction, but it does mean that the victim would reach maximal recovery without the complications of an Energy Cyst. Whereas had the victim been worried about the stock market crashing at the time of the hammer blow from the mugger, those complications of Energy Cyst retention would most likely occur.

Before discussing these complications, I would like to offer several additional ideas which favor Energy Cyst formation and retention. Occasionally I have seen a patient in good health and spirits whose injury was so powerful that it overcame their dissipating abilities. I have also seen Energy Cyst formation in a person in good spirits who is in the recovery phase of a health problem. This person may be physically unable to throw off the force of injury from a present physical trauma. The most common condition which favors Energy Cyst formation and retention, however, is the presence of related or unrelated destructive emotion at the time of injury.

COMPLICATIONS OF ENERGY CYST RETENTION

The complications of Energy Cyst retention depend upon its emotional content, the quantity of energy within the cyst and its location. It seems that the emotional content of an Energy Cyst is capable of entraining the general emotional tone of the whole person. That is, if the Energy Cyst is full of anger, self-righteous indignation and fearful panic—as it might be if the victim were struck on the head during a mugging in broad daylight in Middletown, USA, where it was supposed to be perfectly safe—that person's whole personality might change, becoming quick to anger and always feeling justified in expressing this anger. The victim also might develop certain phobias or paranoid responses when aware of a stranger walking behind him/her. I have seen marked personality changes for the better occur after the release of an Energy Cyst that contained destructive emotion.

The physical/physiological effects of a retained Energy Cyst depend largely upon its potency (quantity of contained energy) and its location. For example, the energy from a fall on the sacrococcygeal complex could penetrate quite easily into the pelvic viscera. In this location, it could cause bladder dysfunction with chronic sphincter control problems, menstrual dysfunction, inability to conceive or maintain a pregnancy, prostatitis and so on, depending upon the exact location of the Energy Cyst. If it didn't penetrate to the viscera, coccydynia would be a good possibility. On the other hand, if it went all the way to the respiratory diaphragm the patient might later begin to notice symptoms of esophageal reflux (heartburn). If it got through the diaphragm, it might penetrate into the cardiac muscle and set the person up for coronary disease at a later date.

The Energy Cyst doesn't produce its full effect right away. The patient's body adapts as best it can; but slowly, over a period of months and years, the seat of the Energy Cyst is compromised in its function. Naturally, the Energy Cyst, by its presence, contributes to the facilitation of the related spinal cord segments. The whole syndrome of segmental facilitation begins.[7]

It was this work with Dr. Karni, our observations of the phenomena related to the model of the Energy Cyst and the observations at the center for autism that set the scene for the other clinical observations I shall now describe.

---

[7] See Appendix A, Facilitated Segment.

CLINICAL OBSERVATIONS

The following observations were made on private patients who were referred to me for consultation as a specialist in manual medicine, biomechanics and osteopathic manipulation techniques. While these individuals were not involved with us as research subjects, I shall nonetheless describe a few of these experiences to provide the flavor of what I was shown.

1.   The first individual was a 38-year-old professional woman, divorced for almost 10 years. She was referred to me by the Department of Psychiatry for consultation about the possibility of structural musculoskeletal causes for persistent and severe pain in the low back and head. She had undergone a vaginal hysterectomy at age 28 under duress from her (then) husband whose insistence was based on the inconvenience tendered him by her PMS and menametarrhagia. He then divorced the patient within a year after the hysterectomy. She had been in psychotherapy for approximately seven of the 10 years that had elapsed since the hysterectomy. Subjects of her focus in her psychotherapy included anger toward men in general, her condition of premature sterility and the probability that the head and low back pain were psychosomatically induced.

During her first visit, I found some somatic dysfunctions of the pelvis and of the upper cervical and occipital regions. The left ilium was posteriorly positioned, the sacrum was torsioned in a compensatory manner and there was compression of the axial-atlanto-occipital complex. Osteopathic and craniosacral therapeutic techniques were applied, and she reported instant relief from pain. (This kind of miraculous "cure" should make you suspicious once you realistically come to grips with your own "therapist's ego." I had met my therapist's ego several years before and was very suspicious that this was only the beginning of our relationship as pain patient and physician.)

After about 10 days the patient called and said that she had about a 50 percent recurrence of the head and back pain. She asked me to see her again. Our next session was about two weeks after the first. This time I treated her in a manner similar to the first but without the miraculous relief of pain that she experienced during the first office visit. She showed me her anger and I knew that psychotherapy had not successfully resolved her negative feelings toward the male gender. She accused me of malingering and intentionally leaving her in pain because I secretly hated women. It was not a pleasant experience, but I had learned over the years that I couldn't take such accusations seriously if I wanted to survive as a healthcare professional.

She insisted on seeing me again in a week's time. (In retrospect, it is obvious that I was encountering the conflict between what we now see as the part of the patient that wants SomatoEmotional Release—I didn't know what SER was at that time—and the part of her that resisted confrontation with the truth. I frequently

quently view this latter part of the patient as the martyred part who says, "Leave well enough alone. I will protect you from this horrible memory realization. My happiness doesn't matter.") At the third visit, the patient reported a little improvement, probably enough to allow her to consciously justify another treatment session with me. Fortunately, I had a graduate student observing during this visit. (It was lucky—if there is such a thing—for me that I did.)

The patient was supine on the treatment table. I had my right hand under her left buttock with my fingers on the sacroiliac. With my left hand, I was moving her left leg up and down gently to evaluate sacroiliac mobility and function. Quite suddenly, her left leg went into flexion at the hip and knee. With no one touching it, the right leg did the same thing. She was in what appeared to be a lithotomy position. I asked the graduate student to support her right leg gently while I did the same with her left leg. (This experience occurred at the same time that we were seeing emotional releases related to body positions at the center for autism. My intuition told me to manage her legs in a way that was similar to the way in which we were obtaining emotional releases by body position with autistic children.) Almost immediately after her legs reached the simulated lithotomy position, we could see a lot of rapid eye movement going on beneath her closed lids. As luck would have it, her purse was in a chair that was within reach of her left hand. The next thing I knew, this nice lady was pummeling my head, neck and right shoulder with her purse. I registered surprise and probably expressed some "expletive deleted"— although I can't tell you exactly what that was. She quickly explained, as though she were a detached third person observer, that the blows were meant for the surgical resident who was leaning too heavily on her left knee. His weight was creating a very severe strain in her back and pelvis. She went on to explain that the anesthesiologist had her neck and her head in a very awkward position of extension that was very painful. She also said to me that this was the occasion of her hysterectomy and that she was completely asleep under the influence of a total anesthesia.

I was taken a bit by surprise by this turn of events. I had done a fair amount of hypnoregression and hypnotherapy in the past and was aware that the nonconscious knows, if not all, damn near all. I was no stranger to the idea that conversation and events during surgical procedures under general anesthesia might be recorded in the nonconscious mind, but all I had done was touch this lady at the left buttock and sacroiliac areas and passively move her left leg to test for sacroiliac mobility— and here she was visualizing her hysterectomy while asleep under a general anesthetic.

My first inclination was to let out an explosive "WOW!" but I contained my enthusiasm, acted as if this were an everyday occurrence and talked with her about how she shouldn't be mad at the surgical resident because he was probably exhausted from the hideously long hours required by the hospital during training. I tried my best to get her to empathize with him, to forgive and forget. The anesthesiologist—who had her head in hyperextension at the atlanto occipital joint and was mightily straining and compressing the upper cervical structures while the protective muscles were rendered essentially helpless by drugs—was more difficult to defend. He had put a tube down her throat, made some conversation about how she was keeping the playpen but losing the baby carriage and was, in general, somewhat less than respectful. I tried to convince her that to stay angry with him, though it might be justified, was hurting her and not him. She accepted this idea to some extent. Re-experiencing the surgery ended—by her choice—just as quickly as it had begun.

I was convinced that we had discovered and dealt with the reasons for her acute anger at men. I thought I understood why the psychotherapy had hit an impasse. I was both over-enthusiastic and incorrect. I set another appointment in a week's time for her. I really wanted to see what was going to happen.

Her next visit was heralded by complaints of nervousness and inability to concentrate, though her pains were appreciably improved. She had not seen her psychotherapist since her first visit with me (which made it about four weeks without psychotherapy.) As she lay on the table in a supine position, the same graduate student was with me. (He had been totally astonished by the events of the last visit. I could not have prevented his attendance at this visit had I wanted to.) This time I made sure there were no potential weapons within her reach and we lifted her legs into the simulated lithotomy position again. (Today, I would not be nearly so directive, but we were eager and had little idea of what we were actually onto as far as therapeutic approach was concerned. There were no ground rules yet.) She (her body) accepted our manual, nonverbal suggestions and her legs went directly to the position as though she were in gynecological stirrups. Her head hyperextended autonomously on her neck into what appeared to be an uncomfortable position, and she immediately began to describe the scene in the operating room as a third party observer. She described in reasonable detail the dissection of the adnexal tissues as the uterus was removed through the vagina. She gave enough anatomical detail to authenticate either her visual image of the experience or her study of surgical anatomy related to the procedures. She concurrently described and reacted in bodily ways to the sensations of intrapelvic tugging and pulling as the surgical procedure continued. Finally, it was done. The uterus was put in a pan and sent to the pathology laboratory. Then she related that the resident who had been leaning on her left leg was told to repair the vaginal incision. "Cuff" was the word she used. She felt this activity as the resident went about the repair process.

The surgeon paid little attention. He passed the time of day in conversation with the surgical nurse. When the resident finished the incisional closure, the surgeon stepped back into the operating area, sat on a stool, looked at the resident's work and remarked that it was a pretty sloppy job. He followed the remark with a statement to the effect that if he had time he would take those sutures out and make the resident do it over—but the next case was ready so he didn't have time.

The patient was furious. I tried to convince her that this probably was the surgeon's way of castigating the resident, that the repair was probably fine and that this castigation of residents and interns is a favorite sport amongst surgeons and other "hot shots." She told me that while this may be true, she had carried an incisional infection for about six months after the surgery and had healed very poorly. She felt that this was one of the things that had prompted her husband to divorce her. Her inability to have satisfactory sex with her husband is what he'd said had driven him to seek satisfaction elsewhere. I tried to convince her that if this was all it had taken to break up her marriage she was probably better off without the relationship. I also tried to convince her that the surgical repair might have been fine but that the nonconsciously received suggestion that it was a second-rate repair might have been enough to slow down and complicate the healing process. (I only wanted to soften the anger.) Finally, what worked was the idea (once again) that being angry with her doctors of 10 years earlier was hurting her and not them. (Anger is a destructive emotion when chronically produced and retained.)

After just a few weeks of what I would now call "bodywork" and "ventilation," she was totally fine. She did not return to psychotherapy. She did lecture to my students about her experiences. She had not had a relationship with a man since her divorce. She was desensitizing, but there was no rush.

2. The second case that crossed my path at about the same time was less dramatic but nearly as instructive as it unfolded. This was a 27-year-old single woman employed as a social worker in New York City. Her mother had been seeing me for chronic leg pain. The daughter had been referred by her mother. The daughter's problem was the gradual onset of increasingly painful debilitation of the left shoulder. I could find very little of a structural nature wrong with the shoulder joint, its related bones, the vertebral column or the ribs. I began the therapeutic positioning work that I was doing with Dr. Karni (but without electrical monitoring). The patient's arm and shoulder went into a position that brought the craniosacral rhythm to an abrupt stop. I waited a few seconds and movement of the arm, shoulder, neck, head and total upper body began. The patient was sitting on the end of the table, and I positioned myself to her left. Slowly, she began to lean way over to the left. Her craniosacral rhythm had not begun yet. She began to topple off the table to her left as though she was going to fall to the floor onto her left shoulder. I managed to support her through this maneuver and allow her to continue her slow descent toward the floor until her left shoulder was perhaps 12 or 14 inches below the level of the table top. Her hips were up on the table. Most of her weight was supported by the table under her left hip and by me under her left shoulder. Here, she stopped her movement. With my back creaking, she remained in this position for at least five minutes (it seemed like an hour) before her craniosacral rhythm began. When the rhythm began, she smiled as she sat upright

on the table and told me she just realized that the shoulder problem was the result of a skiing injury when she was 19 years old.

This single treatment session abated all her symptoms for about three months after her return to New York. She then called and said her shoulder didn't really hurt but was beginning to feel "funny" and was becoming stiff. She returned to my office in Michigan for two visits, one on a Friday and one on the following Monday. During the Friday visit, I simply held her arm and head for a while and very little happened in the sitting position. I asked her to lie supine on the table and again held the left arm and shoulder. She moved a little, her craniosacral rhythm stopped, her shoulder became hot to the touch and she suddenly felt very angry. I asked if she knew why she was angry. After a minute or two, she said that the reason she had fallen while skiing was because another skier cut in front of her. She swerved as a reflexive, self-protective action and she fell, injuring her left shoulder. She was angry with the skier who had cut in front of her. After telling me this, her craniosacral rhythm still did not start. I gently asked her if that were all she was mad about. She waited a few minutes, felt another strong surge of anger and told me that what really made her mad was that the offending skier did not stop to see if she was all right or if she needed some help. After she released this anger, she said she felt light and wonderful. On Monday she still felt fine. I gave her routine osteopathic and craniosacral treatments.

I have seen her about every six months since then, simply because she likes the treatment process. She has released her other problems. She has had absolutely no further shoulder problems since the release of the anger. She has found herself better able to tolerate the frustrations of her profession as a social worker in New York City. (I'm sure her frustrations are many.)

3.   Very soon after the surgical hysterectomy case and between the shoulder case's first and second visits, another surgical memory case came up. (I suppose this happened to properly impress me with the importance of the information to which I had become privy.) This case involved a woman in her mid-twenties who suffered from severe debilitating occipito-frontal headaches. Craniosacral evaluation revealed excessive membranous tension between the glabella of the frontal bone and the midline occiput from the external posterior occipital protuberance (inion, for the people in my age group) inferior to the spine of the axis. I performed some routine craniosacral techniques to loosen the various components of the cranial vault and the floor of the vault. Then I began to V-spread from inion through to glabella. As the V-spread energy began to build, the patient's craniosacral rhythm abruptly stopped. A lot of heat began to radiate from glabella and the midline sutural area between the nasal bones. The patient began to feel a great deal of anger. This angry feeling calmed down as the heat radiation subsided and the V-spread seemed to take its full effect. The craniosacral rhythm recommenced its activity.

I asked the patient if she understood the anger that expressed itself. She told me that it was hard for her to accept, but what came to mind was the surgeon doing her septectomy some years before. As she re-experienced the surgical procedure, the surgeon seemed very angry. She had convinced him to have her put to sleep for the surgery. He didn't like the idea but allowed a general anesthetic against his better judgment.

Here again we have the unconscious recording an event during which the patient was supposed to be asleep. But this case poses other very fascinating questions. Does the emotion of the surgeon enter an Energy Cyst formed in the patient during the surgical procedure? Further, should we consider the surgical procedure a traumatic event able to produce an Energy Cyst? If so, does the anesthetized condition of the patient favor Energy Cyst formation and retention? The implications of these questions are immense.

SOMATOEMOTIONAL RELEASE

The experiences with autistic children, with Dr. Karni and with the three patients described above came together simultaneously. It was as if these experiences had been orchestrated to tell me something. The unavoidable observation that surfaced was that the release of Energy Cysts leads to total body releases that improve mind-body function. It further suggested that we do not need to know about the past injury. All we have to do is place our hands on the patient/client with a gentle sensitive manner, tune into what the body wants to do, follow the movement, counter the effect of gravity, not lead the movement even if we think we know where it is going, ask a few questions or give a little verbal support at critical times—and the body will release not only Energy Cysts but stored up emotions that are contributing to patient discomfort.

With our hands, we were releasing pent-up emotion via the somatic route. Autistic children's affect and sociability improved, angry people became nicer, pain went away and the craniosacral rhythm stopped abruptly at the right time to tell us when we were on the right track. Who in the world would believe this?

But it worked and the results were obvious. People changed, tissues changed, functions improved. (Ultimately, I saw that Kirlian photographs of fingers changed.[8]) Forgotten, repressed incidents came back into conscious awareness as did events recounted from the surgical suite while the patient was asleep. I had no real idea what I was on to, and it was more than a little awe imposing. It was also addictive. I was so intrigued, I couldn't let go of it, and I didn't want to.

We needed a name for this system that would differentiate it clearly from psychosomatic medicine. It clearly wasn't the same, although it dealt with the body-mind interface, it was body-mind not mind-body as was the psychosomatic concept. The name "SomatoEmotional Release" was coined.

I screwed up my courage and taught the first SomatoEmotional Release course in Chicago in 1980. Yesterday's news is obsolete today, but there comes a time when we must stop and document. That's what I'm doing here.

---

[8] During this fast-moving period—using black and white Polaroid film so we could keep track of events as they unfolded—I began taking Kirlian photographs before and after each phase of my private patients' treatments (CranioSacral Therapy and SomatoEmotional Release and sometimes acupuncture). I photographed the right-hand fingertips of all these patients on the same film with my own right-hand fingertips. The energy coronas projecting from both the patient's fingertips and mine appeared markedly changed after treatment.

Chapter II
Energy Cysts and
SomatoEmotional Release

ENERGY CYSTS

The persistent question about Energy Cysts has been whether they can be caused by other than externally induced trauma. That is, can emotion, spiritual conflict, parasites, bacteria, viruses, toxins, malnutrition or genetics induce an Energy Cyst? The answer has to be arbitrary. The concept of the Energy Cyst came from the many observations Dr. Karni and I made regarding the results of externally induced trauma. It was the injection into this body of traumatic energy that resulted in the Energy Cyst as we were introduced to it. I described the Energy Cyst in the preceding chapter. Suffice it here to remind you that it is a localized area of increased entropy that is retained in the body. This increased entropy is disorganized and disruptive energy that the body handles the best way it can.

I do not mean to imply that the only source of a localized area of increased entropy is an external physical trauma. Rather, the sample that presented itself was composed of patients with physical trauma residua that we named "Energy Cysts."

Probably the exclusivity of defining the Energy Cyst as traumatically induced from outside the body is obsolete. I am now sure that areas of increased entropy or Energy Cysts can result from a wide range of problems. It would be more accurate to talk about emotionally induced Energy Cysts, toxically induced Energy Cysts, karmically induced Energy Cysts, virally induced Energy Cysts, traumatically induced Energy Cysts and so on. We must specify the origin or cause of the Energy Cyst as best we can. Traumatically induced Energy Cysts are probably best released by finding and holding the correct therapeutic body position. Other types of Energy Cysts can be released by the direction of energy, intention, SomatoEmotional Release and so on.

Energy Cysts can be discovered in many ways. Occasionally it is as simple as watching the patient point to where it hurts. But don't learn to depend on this method. The patient may be experiencing a referred pain or a secondary joint dysfunction. An Energy Cyst could be obstructing energy flow along an acupuncture meridian anywhere on its course. The pain may then be felt in the related viscera or anywhere else along the course of the meridian. You just can't depend on pain to show you where the Energy Cyst is located.

Arcing is probably the best method for localizing the Energy Cyst. Arcing is another of those concepts that came out of our research as Karni and I attempted to understand what I was doing when I evaluated and treated a patient. I was doing intuitive arcing intuitively. It remained for Dr. Karni to force me to try to describe what I was doing and for him to make good physics sense from my descriptions.

After much observation and discussion, we decided I was perceiving with my hands the energies that apparently emanate from an "active lesion" which is really an Energy Cyst. We applied the name "arcing" because it best described the sense that therapists/facilitators get through their hands as they tune in to the energy of the Energy Cyst or any other active lesion.

It is as though the Energy Cyst is at the center point of an infinite number of concentric globes that are vibrating rotationally. Any specific point on the surface of any of the globes describes a small arc as though it is the free end of a pendulum (the radius of the globe) swinging to and fro, with the pendulum's central attachment at the center of the globe. The pendulum swing ignores gravity. Since the therapist/facilitator has two hands, in an arcing evaluation, each hand perceives a slightly different arc, because the distance from the Energy Cyst is different for each hand. (Occasionally the central focus is equidistant from each hand. This can get confusing; just move your hands to different positions to end the confusion.) The problem is to project from each hand where the common central attachment for the two pendula is located or where the projected radii of the two arcs would meet. These globes can be felt on or off the body. The number of globes is infinite. Therefore, it doesn't matter at what distance your hands are from the Energy Cyst, you will feel the "arcing" activity.

If you will think in two dimensions for a moment, these energy waves given off by the Energy Cyst might be considered analogous to the concentric ripples or interference waves given off when you drop a pebble into the smooth surface of a pond. The natural smooth wave activity of the pond might be considered as the craniosacral rhythm. The waves of interference superimposed on the pond surface by the disruption of the pebble may be seen as the phenomenon we are calling arcing.

The rotational, rhythmical vibrating rate, in my experience, has been consistently more rapid than the rate of the craniosacral rhythm. It also has been slower than the heart rate. It seems not to be affected by the patient/client's breathing.

The arcing system of Energy Cyst discovery and location has not changed appreciably since Dr. Karni and I developed the model in 1976. You can place your hands anywhere on the body and perceive, by arcing, the presence of an Energy Cyst anywhere in the body if the effect is not dampened out of your perception by distance and perhaps density of the medium through which the energy must travel.

As you place your hands in different positions on and off the patient's body, you can begin to zero in on the Energy Cyst by finding hand positions that give you arcs with smaller and smaller radii. When you are directly over the central focus, the Energy Cyst, for all the arcs you have experienced, the sensation is as though you are above a pinwheel that rotates a short distance in one direction, then in the other. The rate of vibration is variable from one Energy Cyst to the next, within the parameters of heart rate at the high end and craniosacral rhythm rate at the low end.[9]

---

[9] See *CranioSacral Therapy*, pp. 244 – 245 and 249 – 250 and *CranioSacral Therapy II, Beyond the Dura*, p. 216, for a more thorough description of arcing concepts and techniques. (The best way to learn to do arcing evaluation is during CranioSacral Therapy Level II workshop practice sessions.)

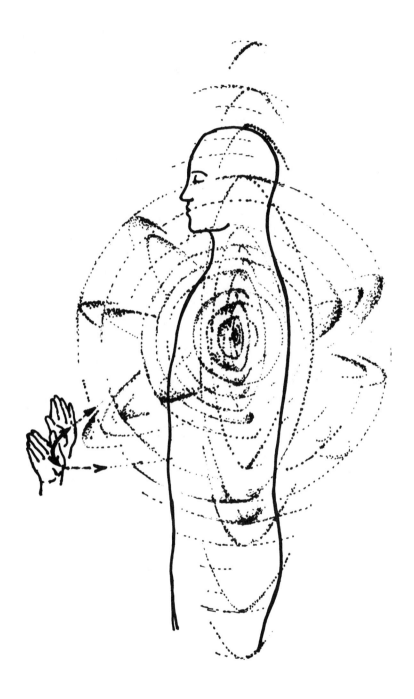

Hands palpate the rotationally vibrating energy created by the Energy Cyst
located in the mid-thorax. Arcing can be done on and off the body. See text.
Illustration II – 1

As you all know by now, Fascial Glide and symmetry/asymmetry of craniosac-ral movement can also be used to locate Energy Cysts,[10] but these methods will also locate any other cause of fascial restriction. The restriction of movement might be from adhesions left from a previously active problem or could be due to muscle imbalance—or even a key or wallet in the pocket. So, do not over-interpret your findings. Arcing is probably the most reliable method of discovery of active prob-lems including Energy Cysts.

Palpation of obstructed acupuncture meridia may also lead you to an Energy Cyst that may be causing an obstruction. An obstructed meridian could also be the residuum of a previous problem that is no longer active, however. If you do feel an empty or a very full meridian, it is worth the time to manually trace that meridian along its course to discover whether an Energy Cyst is present. If you do discover an Energy Cyst, you will feel the arcing activity as you approach it and may well feel heat and other qualitative sensations related to a focus of increased energy.

If you practice Chinese pulse diagnosis, it is fun to locate a meridian problem first by the pulses. Then palpate the meridian in its entirety (as far as possible) in search of Energy Cyst blockage. If you find it, correct it as you monitor the pulse. As the Energy Cyst is released, the Chinese pulse will change toward normal. If it is physically impossible to monitor pulses while you release the Energy Cyst, second best is to recheck the pulse after Energy Cyst release is completed. You'll miss the process, but at least you'll feel the effect of your treatment upon another bodily system.

Since our original work, my clinical observations have repeatedly shown that the Energy Cyst can cause dysfunction in the form of pain, but it also can contrib-ute to the formation of Facilitated Segments.[11] In this way it may actually contrib-ute to specific visceral disease in the future. The number of internal organ prob-lems that can be caused either by Energy Cysts directly or by Energy Cyst contri-bution to Segmental Facilitation is inestimable.

Energy Cysts may retain negative emotions and seem to somehow entrain the total person. I have seen many examples of Energy Cyst-retained anger which seemed to cause the total personality to operate in an angry mode. This is also true of other destructive emotions such as guilt and fear.

I have also seen Energy Cysts with significant placement cause energy center/chakra dysfunction. I have had patients who spent years working on one or an-other energy center only to have it become dysfunctional soon after it is corrected.

---

[10] See *CranioSacral Therapy*, Chapter XIV, and *CranioSacral Therapy II, Beyond the Dura*, Chapter IV, for all other methods of whole body evaluation used in CranioSacral Therapy. Hands-on application of these techniques is part of the CranioSacral Therapy Level II Workshops.

[11] See Appendix A, Facilitated Segment.

Patients/clients may begin to blame themselves for having a spiritual defect that prevents them from achieving good and lasting chakra function.[12] Usually this self-blame is unwarranted, and the problem is corrected by release of an Energy Cyst.

Dr. Karni and I originally hypothesized—and I continue to feel—that the presence of an Energy Cyst disrupts the normal flow of micro-currents and energies within the fascial system. We intended to investigate this concept further. Dr. Karni made reservations with a friend of his for the shielded room at the Massachusetts Institute of Technology. Here, we were going to attempt to measure, or at least illustrate with instruments, the patterns of flow of micro-currents in the human body by mapping the magnetic fields created by these currents. Dr. Karni, at Michigan State University on a visiting professorship for three years, was called back to Israel. He was unable to obtain a renewal of his visiting faculty status and the research was interrupted. Therefore we could not complete this phase of our work. We did make some attempts to measure and map the magnetic fields at Oakland University in Pontiac, Michigan, but their shielded room was not of the quality required.

I have not yet found a more effective method for the treatment of the Energy Cyst than to follow the body to its individual preferred position of release, the therapeutic position. The patient's body always seems to know best what it should do. A problem or obstacle to treatment may be presented by a part of the patient that may wish to maintain status quo. As therapists/facilitators, we must identify the part of the patient that wants to be relieved of the Energy Cyst and support it without offending that part which wants the status quo; both are trying to do the best they can for the patient.

This kind of conflict within the patient/client as it relates to an Energy Cyst usually shows itself as rapid, repetitive body movement that takes you to the edge of the therapeutic position and then speeds past it. When this kind of rapid movement occurs, I suggest that you follow it a few cycles so you are familiar with the movement pattern. Then slow it down. Become a slight inhibitory factor. Don't stop the movement; just make the body part in question work to move your hands along with it. When you get to the edge of the therapeutic position, the craniosacral rhythm will stop suddenly. When this sudden stop occurs, don't let the body part move past it. Hold it there and it will feel as though it drops into a "notch." You now have the therapeutic position.

In my mind, I characterize these rapid, repetitive movements as a manifestation of the internal debate between the patient/client parts. One part is saying, "Let's get rid of this nuisance, this Energy Cyst." The opposing part is saying, "Let's

---

[12] See *CranioSacral Therapy II, Beyond the Dura,* pp. 229 – 230, for a description of chakras and how to treat them.

leave well enough alone. Why stir things up?" You, as the therapeutic facilitator, are aligning your energy with the former of these two parts, saying, "If you want to get rid of this nuisance, I'll help you right now."

Another image that comes to mind when it seems as if you are nearly to the therapeutic position—but not quite—is that the patient/client's nonconscious is testing your dedication and skill. Dedication testing is carried out to see if you are patient and dedicated enough to go through the wild goose chase to get to the meat of the matter and stay with it. Skill-testing is carried out to see if you have the know-how to deal with the problem and its sequelae once the Energy Cyst is dislodged and the release of its contents begins. In short, the patient/client's nonconscious is testing your intent.

SOMATOEMOTIONAL RELEASE

To describe SomatoEmotional Release (S.E.R.) on any given day is a most difficult task. Every day that I work with this process, it changes. What I wrote yesterday is obsolete today. I learn something new each time I work with it. There are, however, two analogies or models for the S.E.R. process that seem to persist in my imagination. I share these models with you in the sincere hope that this sharing will be helpful as your S.E.R. concept develops and grows.

THE TREE MODEL

In the first of these two models, I see the S.E.R. process as the trunk of a tree of which CranioSacral Therapy (CST) is the root system. The roots are well grounded in the earth, just as CST concepts are firmly grounded in the structures and functions of the bones of the skull, sacrum and coccyx; the sutures and their contents; the meningeal membrane system, especially the dura mater; the ventricular system of the brain; the choroid system; the arachnoid and venous sinus systems; the cerebrospinal fluid system; and the mechanisms described in the PressureStat model. As nodes on this root system which furnish information, we might see the techniques used in whole body diagnosis and in the diagnosis and treatment of facilitated segments.

The (CST) roots converge to form the tree trunk which is S.E.R.. This trunk acts as a two-way conduit that conducts water and nutrients up to the branches and leaves from the roots and energy (as sugar from photosynthesis) down to the root system from the leaves. The main branches coming off the S.E.R. trunk include such things as therapeutic imagery, therapeutic dialogue, mind-body/body-mind integration, self awareness, self-clearing, channeling, spiritual growth, out of body experiences, past life experiences and so on.

Energy Cysts (in this model) may be considered components of the trunk (S.E.R.). Allowed to follow its natural course, Energy Cyst release will ultimately if not immediately lead to S.E.R., which in turn conducts the unified patient/client-facilitator complex to the most skyward of the branches. The product of these highest branches and their leaves is conducted back to the root (CST) system via the trunk (S.E.R.).

In this model, the interdependence between the root system (CST), the trunk (S.E.R.) and all the branches and leaves (the long list of branches to which S.E.R. leads is given, at least in part, above) is clear and irrefutable. Without the (CST) root system, the (S.E.R.) trunk would not exist. It is the (S.E.R.) trunk that has led us to the most exalted of facilitative and healing modes that we see as branches of various sizes and shapes.

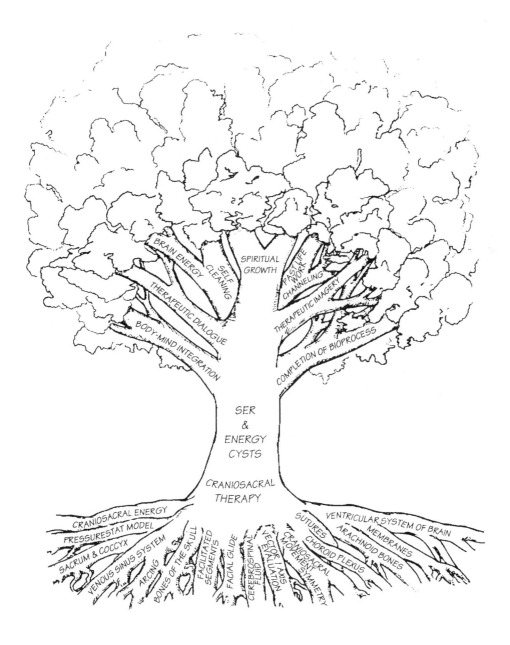

The tree model shows the crucial connecting function of S.E.R. in relation to other therapeutic modalities used by CranioSacral Therapists.

Illustration II – 2

BRAIN GENERATOR MODEL

The second analogy (or model) that just won't go away has your brain as the creator/generator of a multitude of very different, precise and specific energies to which various body parts resonate. These resonating body parts include everything from your viscera to your ions. All types of tissues, fluids, molecules and the like are included. As the extraencephalic body parts begin to respond and resonate, each to its specific and individual type of energy, they send messages back to the brain to let it know the brain's message has been received and is being acted upon.

These messages from the brain might be intended for white blood cells, telling them to activate because bacterial aliens have made entry into the body. It could be that the brain is sending messages to tell your liver to increase bile production to clear a fat soluble toxin. Or it might be a message to constrict the blood vessels around a snake bite to slow the spread of venom.

We know that nerves and hormones conduct information to and from end organs, but many things that happen every day are very difficult to explain solely using the concepts of nerve and blood borne messages. Why not consider the idea that the brain can and does produce specific energies that cause specific body parts to resonate in specific ways? This might explain the use of healing energies, both autonomous and from external sources. It may explain how you, as a therapeutic facilitator, can activate the patient/client's self-healing mechanisms.

If this is true, think for a moment about the potential of the work that CranioSacral Therapy does to facilitate brain function and improve the internal milieu in which the brain must function. Considered from this point of view, it becomes totally reasonable that CranioSacral Therapy can help the patient/client significantly in the battle against anything from flu to cancer, hyperkinesis to endogenous depression. Why not? CranioSacral Therapy vitalizes the brain. This vitalization may enable the brain to send more precise, specifically correct and powerful energy messages in a more appropriate and efficient manner.

The extraencephalic body components that receive and resonate to energy messages from the brain may be rendered dysfunctional—to almost any degree from very little to completely. The dysfunction may be caused by the presence of anything that interferes with or distorts the energetic messages sent by the brain. Or it can be caused by anything that impairs the body components' abilities to resonate or confirm receipt of the message. Energy Cysts seem likely causes of interference. They may be located anywhere in the feedback loop.

An energy message en route from brain to peripheral body component may be distorted or even obliterated during an encounter with an Energy Cyst. A distortion in the energy message could mean that it is not received by its intended body component or it could mean that the body component responds to an incorrect message. This response could mean that the body component may do something that is out of harmony with total body function. This could contribute to self-destructive processes such as we see in leukemia and the autoimmune disease groups.

An Energy Cyst also may be located within an intended extraencephalic body component resonator. In this location, the Energy Cyst could interfere with that component's ability to resonate correctly, if at all. Or it could interfere with that body component's ability to send the message back to the brain that the original brain to body component message had been received. Here, the brain, not realizing that the body component is complying with the original energetic message, continues to send out more of the same. The resonating extraencephalic body component may then continue to act beyond the desired level. This could result in over-responsiveness and the wearing out of organs or response mechanisms. An Energy Cyst that intercepts and changes or nullifies the energy messages sent out by the resonating body component also could cause hyper-response. And certainly, an Energy Cyst within the brain could render the whole system dysfunctional.

Interference in the system, put forth in this model, can be caused by the Energy Cyst as Dr. Karni and I originally thought of it as induced by external trauma or by comparable localized areas of increased entropy (energetic disorganization) that we can call Energy Cysts—caused by emotion, bacteria, viruses, toxins, electromagnetic pollutants, radiation and so on. Loci of energetic disorganization that have come about by any mechanism can, indeed, interfere with how intact the delicate energy message loops remain that exist between the brain creator/generator and the extraencephalic body component resonators.

Energy Cyst Release and SomatoEmotional Release serve to help clear the body and its immediate energy fields of extraneous energies and interferences that possess the potential for disruption of this system. Clearly, Vector/Axis Alignment and Integration and chakra work also become significant approaches in this model. I consider this model as another branch from the S.E.R. tree trunk.[13, 14]

---

[13] Since writing this, I have had the privilege to read *The Dark Side of the Brain* in which authors Harry Oldfield and Roger Coghill expound a similar theory. Well worth a read, it is published by Element Books Ltd., Great Britain.

[14] Research physicist Neil Mohon likened the system described in this model to the remote control systems used in everything from model boats to those used by NASA to control space shots.

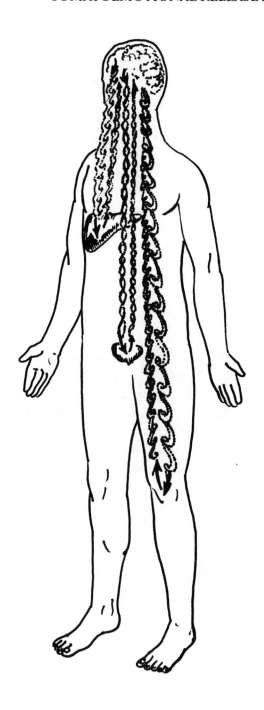

Signals to extracephalic body parts originate in the brain and are received by specific body parts. Receipt is acknowledged. This communication is by energy wave signals, an addition to nerve and molecular communication. See text.

Illustration II – 3

INITIATION OF S.E.R.

The longer I practice in the system of therapeutic facilitation, the more I realize the power of intention. The intention I use so often is the intent to support whatever that patient/client's inner wisdom[15] wants to do at that time. So my first intention is to let the patient/client know that whatever they want to do is okay with me. This is transmitted nonverbally through my initial touch. We will talk about many things. Our voices may be saying one thing and our touch communicating something entirely different. As the integration within the patient/client between conscious and nonconscious awareness progresses, we may very gently and with great sensitivity begin to verbalize that which our touch communication has been considering since we began the session.

In practical terms, this means that when I first put my hands on a patient/client, I say to him/her silently, "If you want to do CranioSacral Therapy that's what we'll do; show me where to begin. If you have a pressing issue with an Energy Cyst that's okay. We'll do that. Show me where you would like me to be. If SomatoEmotional Release is what you want to do, just start and I'll be with you. Go ahead and image all you want to. Please share those images with me. Perhaps I can help you understand what they are trying to tell you. We'll dialogue anytime you want to. Just let me know when you are ready. Whatever you think is the best way to come toward resolution of this problem is okay with me. Let's do it." And so on.

It is wonderful the way the patient/client's body then begins to respond to your offering of help. You don't have to say a word until their body tells you to start talking—but I repeat, small talk is a wonderful distracter; it helps the body get past the mind's defenses.

It has been at least three years since I have put a patient in the sitting or standing position to initiate a SomatoEmotional Release process. I touch each one of them with silent statements about my intention. Their body transmits my touch message to their nonconscious or higher intelligence, higher self, whatever you prefer to call it. The touch, if sincerely well-intentioned and non-threatening, establishes a bond of trust between you and the patient/client's nonconscious (perhaps the conscious too, but I'm not as concerned with conscious awareness at the beginning). Once you establish the trust and intended understanding, you may be tested a time or two. Sometimes I believe wild goose chases are activated to see if we really are willing to follow. Sometimes confrontations erupt to test your ego stake in the process that you are offering to work through with the patient/client. Sometimes you will get mixed messages that perhaps are testing your ability to follow

---

[15] The concepts of intent, touch and inner wisdom are thoroughly discussed in Chapter V.

patiently and adapt or that may truly represent intended conflict within the patient/client, for example. You may be asked to prove your willingness to subordinate your ego in many ways. If you fail the test, all is not lost, however. It simply sets the process back a little—or perhaps all the way back to square one.

If, after you establish trust, a standing or sitting position for SomatoEmotional Release is desirable, you will sense it as this information comes in through your hands to your conscious awareness. The patient/client's body will very subtly begin to move into a position. Do not disbelieve. If the craniosacral rhythm stops and the patient/client's body seems to want to stand on its head, go with it. Trust what your hands tell you. If you see an end position in your mind's eye, it is probably correct. Nonetheless, wait for the patient/client's body to take you there. Remember, nothing is too weird—but wait for the patient/client to take you there.

There are a few exceptions. When you see an end position clearly and persistently and the patient/client seems unable to get there, you may lead/direct to that place. The picture you are seeing probably is being put there by the patient/client's nonconscious. If you have left your baggage at the door, it may be telling you that you will need to offer some leadership to get past the obstacles.

A good example of this situation wherein I had to direct the patient past a significant block to a strange place that challenged our ability to trust came up during an Advanced CranioSacral Therapy class. The subject in question was a fortyish woman therapist who had been repeating the same SomatoEmotional Release process over and over. I intervened to break the repetitive cycle. As this challenge was put into her system, I began to realize that the patient needed to re-enact her birth process. Her repetitive cycle was apparently symbolic of her moving in space before she entered the product of conception in her mother's uterus. Something was holding her back from entering the fetus that was already implanted. We helped her enter the fetus. Then her great fear of the delivery became apparent. There was also perceptible frustration with the way that her obstetrical delivery had occurred. I began to see clearly that I was to be the cervix located in her mother's body. The patient just couldn't get to it; she was really stuck. The image became more and more clear to me, so I finally decided to act on the image that was in my mind. If the image was wrong, we would have wasted some time and would have to start over; if the image was right, perhaps we could move past this "stuckness." I enacted what I saw in my mind's eye.

I put the patient on my shoulder with the help of the rest of the therapeutic group while I stood on the treatment table. I made a "cervix" with my hands. We held the patient head down with her pelvis on my shoulder and her feet and legs up toward the ceiling. I really concentrated on being that cervix. Her head crowned through the ring I formed with my thumbs and index fingers. As her head was "delivered" through my hands, I—the cervix—had to dilate more. I formed the cervical ring with my arms. First her shoulder began to pass through. Then came her arm, then the other shoulder and the other arm. I maintained my arms as the cervical part of the birth canal; the four participating therapeutic facilitator assistants supported her body from above and guided her down through my arms (the "cervical passage") until her whole body was delivered and we were holding her in the air suspended by her ankles. The process took well over 15 minutes. We had to go slowly and painstakingly; we had to be sensitive to every detail. It was very hard physical work. We did not want to have to repeat it because we had overlooked some detail due to our fatigue or impatience.

Her "guides" seemed to have been with us. (See Chapter VII.) We seem to have followed the process correctly as it was laid out before us. The subject was very different after we completed the session. Today she is much happier and freer. (She sent me a Mother's Day card thanking me for being a good cervix.)

In this case I had to decide where to intervene upon a blocked repetitive process. I had to trust intuition even when it carried me into the ridiculously sublime transition of being a maternal cervix.

When you keep getting an image or impression, there may come a time when you have to take the situation at hand and act upon your image to get past an obstacle. Be sure that you recognize that you are leading. Try to be sure that you have left your baggage out of the treatment session and that what you are going to act upon belongs to the patient/client and not to you or someone else in the room. Proceed with your direction but always be willing to recognize that if it begins to feel that way, your direction may be inappropriate. Don't be afraid to follow an incorrect process to a reasonable end point; accept the idea that you may have erred and start over. Don't let your ego involvement prevent you from accepting your error. I believe that it is important that you follow the error to a gentle ending point. Don't just stop and say something insensitive such as, "Aw merde, this is wrong; we have to start over." Be soft and say something like, "Well, that was part of it. Let's go back and see if we have missed anything."

MULTIPLE FACILITATOR S.E.R.

Until a few years ago, I believed that a competent individual therapeutic facilitator could do S.E.R. as well as a group of therapeutic facilitators; it would just take longer to get to the end result. I did concede that in a few instances, such as the example in which I was the maternal cervical canal, it might be impossible to physically re-enact an experience without extra muscle power from assistant therapeutic facilitators or just sensitive and willing helpers who were willing to follow directions. I also preached the gospel that said that when it was physically impossible to positionally simulate an experience we could image through it satisfactorily.

In retrospect, I believe I was trying very hard to keep S.E.R. within the practical grasp of those solo practitioners who wished to study and use this method. I continue to be convinced that most S.E.R. cases can be done by the unassisted, ego-subordinated and skilled therapeutic facilitator. It takes more time, greater patience and requires the improvisational ingenuity that comes largely with time and experience in S.E.R. work.

Still, it has been shown to me in both the Advanced CranioSacral Therapy classes and in the Brain and Spinal Cord Dysfunction Center that there are times when the depth of release probably cannot be achieved as well by a solo S.E.R. therapeutic facilitator as it can be by a well-coordinated group of therapists/facilitators acting as extra energy sources, extra hands and extra brains. In the Advanced CranioSacral Therapy work, we now focus more and more on the importance of developing skill excellence as an assistant therapeutic facilitator.

This means that as the assistant you become an extension of the therapeutic facilitator who is conducting/orchestrating the session with the patient/client's nonconscious. (As the assistant you become a part of a loop.) You become a perceptual auxiliary station for the conductor, feeding perceptions and sensations to that conductor. You also blend with the patient/client to better perceive and transmit information to your conductor. On occasion, insights may come into your conscious awareness that you will share with the conductor, but you will not act upon them without being instructed to do so by your conductor. This situation of conductor with assistants significantly enhances the conductor's (therapeutic facilitator in charge) energy, perceptual ability and intuitive insight as well as intellectual potential. The level of enhancement depends upon his/her skill and sensitivity levels.

Where there is an experienced group of therapists/facilitators working in harmony under the direction of an open conductor, the depth of penetration and blending with a patient/client is greatly increased. I do not believe that this depth of work can always be attained by a solo therapeutic facilitator, even over a protracted period. And so, I must revise my original stance on this issue. I encourage you to spend perhaps one afternoon or evening per week working group style with your more difficult patients/clients.

COMPLETION OF BIOLOGICAL PROCESS

As time has passed and experiences have been gained, a most fascinating concept has been formulating. It seems that repeatedly in the SomatoEmotional Release process we are asked to complete obstetrical delivery processes from both the infant's and the mother's point of view. It is also very common to find the SomatoEmotional Release process completing a death transition or other transition process.

Perhaps I use the word "complete" incorrectly. The processes of delivery and transition to which I refer have been completed in a pragmatic way but they seem not to have been completed in a qualitative, satisfactory way as judged by some bioinstinct, morphogenetic energy field, gene, chromosome, DNA or whatever: By this, I mean that a naturally planned or predetermined process has somehow been thwarted.

I first began to see this occur clearly with Caesarian Section-delivered patients. There is a significantly larger number of craniosacral system dysfunctions in these Caesarian Section-delivered patients/clients that, unless corrected, seem to persist throughout life. (See Appendix I *CranioSacral Therapy* [Volume I], Upledger and Vredevoogd, "The Relationship of CranioSacral Examination Findings in Grade School Children with Developmental Problems," Upledger.) I attributed this finding to the sudden fluid pressure change that occurs when a uterus is quickly incised, and the mother's water has not been broken previously (as happens in most Caesarian Section deliveries). The baby is subject to a very rapid decompression (from higher intrauterine fluid pressure to lower extrauterine pressure). And make no mistake, this is a rapid pressure change. I have seen amniotic fluid squirt out of a uterine incision several inches into the air. This is analogous to a diver coming to the water's surface very rapidly from a significant depth. In infants it seems reasonable that the delicate infant membranes that are such an intricate part of the craniosacral system may be strained or even slightly torn at this sudden pressure change. Adaptation to this rapid decompression is a lot to ask of an infant, not only in the membranous boundaries of the semiclosed hydraulic craniosacral system but also in any of the fluid compartments. It is a tribute to the resiliency of the infant that more damage is not done more often.

This seems a valid explanation for the significantly higher number of craniosacral system dysfunctions found in Caesarian Section babies as described in the above referenced research report. This explanation occurred to me in 1978 as we were collecting data. A few years later it also became apparent that Caesarian Section babies, in addition to being rapidly decompressed, miss their first, total-body treatment. This has been shown to me by several patients/clients re-experiencing the vaginal delivery process via SomatoEmotional Release, over and over again, as they twist their way through the process. Cranial vault, cervical, thoracic, lumbar and pelvic releases occur. Pain sources become apparent and then often disappear.

As the head passes through the birth canal, the bones overlap and then the cranial vault slowly expands as the head presents. In normal birth, this is all done in good time if the doctor or midwife is not too eager to get the process over.

(All this became extremely clear to me as I reprocessed my own vaginal delivery. I shall never forget my sense of the doctor wanting to pull me out. He pulled whenever he had a chance to get a finger hold on my head or my mouth or my chin, etc. It was clear to me that I wanted to be born, but I wanted to go slowly, especially in certain phases of the process because I could feel my body being correctly adjusted by the birth canal pressures, angulations, movements and so on. I screamed silently to this well-meaning doctor, "Please leave me right here until this is finished. Then let me be pushed out as it was meant to be, not pulled out as you think it ought to be." During my session, I was able, with the help of my own therapeutic facilitator, to modify this part of my delivery to serve my personal needs and desires. The modification has really helped my body.)

In any case, the Caesarian Section infant is cheated out of this passage through the birth canal that I now view as a very important part of the preparation for extrauterine life. Now, I thought, I surely had the total answer to the increased incidence of craniosacral system dysfunctions seen in Caesarian Section children. Wrong again, Upledger.

Over the past several years, it has since been shown to me that there is a programmed process put into place for both mother and fetus when the pregnancy begins. The fetus is supposed to go—by some direction of instinct, genes, energy fields or some other reference that we don't yet know—through its intrauterine development. It will then be pushed out of the uterus through a specially-designed birth canal on a therapeutic trip in preparation for extrauterine life. When something such as a Caesarian Section or forceps delivery interrupts or distorts this naturally-intended process, there seems to occur some sort of retained biological frustration that can manifest in a variety of ways. Most of these ways have to do with qualitative function or chronic pain. When, during the SomatoEmotional Release process, the obstetrical delivery is completed as nature intended, the sense of biological frustration or incompleteness of process disappears and the general function of the patient/client significantly improves; pains disappear, obsessive compulsive behaviors lose potency and so on.

The same seems true of the mother. When a pregnancy begins, it is as though a computerized process is put into motion. This process is complete only when vaginal delivery is done and mother-child bonding has occurred. When the natural process is thwarted by Caesarian Section, general anesthesia, forceps delivery and/ or not having bonded, there is an incompleteness attached to the biological process that has been set in motion by the implantation of the fertilized egg. Again, this biological incompleteness can manifest in many ways. One that has become apparent is the inability to conceive again. Other manifestations include various endocrine, nervous, behavioral and pain problems. Once this biological program is carried to completion via the SomatoEmotional Release process, many of these dysfunctions and symptoms seem to correct themselves automatically.

In addition to the birth process being programmed by nature to process through certain steps for both mother and child, it seems that the process of dying is programmed. This concept derives from two general categories of experience: The multitude of SomatoEmotional Release experiences that involve past lives in which the patient/client seems to regress for the purpose of dying again, usually doing so more acceptably in the re-experience of the process. I'm sure that most of you in your SomatoEmotional Release work have been with patients/clients who have experienced or fantasized a past life and a frustration with that death. They carry with them a set of symptoms into this life. These symptoms disappear spontaneously once the frustration, anger, guilt or fear from the past life or death in question is resolved. It is as though the death process of the past life is incomplete. I used to think that the only significant factor was the resolution of the destructive emotion or sense of frustration with which they died. Now I'm thinking a little differently. The resolution is not only a question of forgiveness, it also involves a qualitatively correct completion of that process of dying. The dying is intended to be the qualitatively correct completion of the past lifetime.

Death is part of life and nature says it must be completed properly. Perhaps part of that completion process is to review what we have done with the lifetime. Take stock of it. Evaluate what we have been shown. See what we have learned. Accept death as the end of another chapter in our existence. Once this is done, there seems no need to carry the sense of incompleteness with us any longer.

Second is my experience in the "here and now" with people who are lingering before death. They seem stuck. Everyone can see that the person is dying, but they are taking so long to do it, with so much resistance, pain and suffering. Once a resolution with life is reached, they are able to go ahead and complete the process. I'm sure if they die before they are ready, they will carry the biological incompleteness with them into a next life or into eternity. This incompleteness may serve to frustrate them until the life is brought to completion by a proper death process.

I was beginning to be shown this lesson when I was an intern in 1963 – 64. I came onto the night shift to be confronted with a patient who had just returned from abdominal surgery. He was a man who had come from Poland. He was in his mid-forties. He had cancer of the pancreas which had spread throughout his abdomen. The surgery had been an exploratory procedure. When the surgeons saw all the cancer growth, they decided to just close him up. They were unable to stop all the internal bleeding.

Neither the man nor his family had any idea that he was going to die. I was told to keep him alive as long as I could, to notify his wife and family who were not at the hospital and to obtain the last rites from a priest. The patient had two units of whole blood running, one into each of his arms. He also had IVs running into each of his legs.

I got acquainted with him both personally and physiologically. It was obvious that he could die at any moment. As I watched, his blood pressure dropped. He lost consciousness. I put some Aramine (a vasopressor to raise his blood pressure) through his IV tubing and he regained consciousness. He smiled and said, "I almost died, didn't I?" I didn't want to say "Yes," but I did.

How could I lie to this man? He asked me whether he could get better. I told him he was riddled with cancer and that he was bleeding inside. I told him that I didn't see how he could get better, but …. I told him I would be with him all night and would do my best to do what he wanted.

He wanted to say good-bye to his wife who was at home and he wanted the last rites from a Catholic priest. He went unconscious again as his blood pressure took another dive. I gave him another dose of Aramine. He came back, smiled and said, "Good work." I had never been so complimented in my life.

I quickly called his home. (The telephone was about 10 yards from the door of his room.) His brother answered the phone. I told him what was going on. He said he would be at the hospital within an hour with the wife (who didn't speak English).

Then the nurse called me back into the room. He was unconscious again and his blood pressure was way down. Aramine had worked twice so I thought I would try it a third time. I did and he came back. I'll never forget how he looked me in the eye and said, "I almost died that time." I told him that his wife and brother were on the way in and that I was going to try for a priest now. I asked him to please hang on until we got all this stuff done. By now, it was after 11 p.m. It was winter in Detroit and blizzard-like. I called three parishes before I found a priest who said he would come in and give this man his last rites.

I went back in the room to find him fading again; more Aramine brought him back again. The priest came in before the wife and brother. He gave last rites and I could see relief on the patient's face. The priest was just leaving when the wife and brother arrived. I gave the patient a little more Aramine so that he could talk to his wife and brother. I left the room. In a few minutes, the brother came out and asked what I could do; his brother was unconscious. I went into the room with the idea that I would let him die this time.

His wife looked pleadingly into my eyes. I gave him more Aramine. He came back again and said, "Thank you. I want a little more time, if you can do it, to make my wife feel better." Feeling as though I was in Rod Serling's other dimension, I left the room totally confused about my values and the position I found myself in. His wife came out shortly and gave me that look again. I went in and gave more Aramine. He came back but this time he said, "I can go now, you don't need to bring me back anymore." I didn't and he left about 45 minutes later for the last time.

I thought about that experience for quite awhile. He knew when he had brought his process to completion. He had not been forewarned that this was to be the last night of this incarnate life. It took him a few hours to get it all in order, reach a resolution and allow the process to go to completion. Today, I'm sure that had he died before receiving the last rites or before talking with his brother and his wife, he would have died prematurely. Even though it was a question of only a couple of hours, had he died prematurely, the process would perhaps have been thwarted. He would have died frustrated and angry—and perhaps carried these destructive feelings into a next life.

Part of our work as therapists/facilitators is to help prepare the patient/client for a nice, clean entry into the next life. I really believe those few hours of meaningful life extension made a great deal of difference for him.

On the other side of the coin, it may be a physiological "stuckness" that interferes with the death process. An osteopath with whom I am very close sent me a letter about an experience she had that said it all. She had a patient in the hospital who was dying of lung cancer. She was dying in great distress and with great effort. My friend says that she simply touched the patient's cranial vault. The vault was in marked extension and stuck there. My friend then exaggerated the extension and a release occurred. The cranial vault went into a large flexion cycle. The patient smiled, took one very deep, relaxed breath and died with a smile on her face. Perhaps her physiological dying process got stuck.

There are probably many non-death transitions that we try to make but are obstructed somehow. SomatoEmotional Release can often help bring these processes to completion as nature intended. When we complete natural processes the way they are intended, I believe we are then free to move on in a more constructive way.

Since the writing of this section on completion of the biological process, yet another process comes to my attention as a candidate for this category of phenomenon. This process is motherhood. There is much concern about career, profession, biological clocks and motherhood in these times of birth control and abortion. For your consideration, please allow me to offer the idea that the first menstrual cycle with ovulation may trigger a biological process that will not go to completion until pregnancy, delivery and maternal bonding have occurred. If no children are born to the woman in question, the reproductive process is frustrated and incomplete and may foster a variety of symptoms.

In a 1990 Advanced CranioSacral Therapy Class, we were blessed with two women as participants who were agonizing over the problems of motherhood versus career advancement. In both cases we managed, as therapeutic facilitators, to do S.E.R. with therapeutic imagery and dialogue in such a way that the motherhood process went to completion—at least in their fantasies.

In both cases, these experiences seemed to satisfy the process which had been set into motion at menarche but which was not completed, even once as they neared the magic age of 40. Imaging through conception, pregnancy, delivery and bonding seemed to resolve the agony related to the question of motherhood versus career and professional advancement.

"Will wonders never cease," my mother used to say.

SOME NEW EXPERIENCES

During 1989, two very significant lessons were presented to me. I'll share them and you can make of them what you wish. I know they are not complete yet, but I wouldn't feel good about holding them back until I know more about them. Both incidents occurred while I was working in our Brain and Spinal Cord Dysfunction Center with patients/clients who were there for our intensive two-week program.

1. There was a male patient in his thirties. He had been one of the victims of a Los Angeles freeway sniper. The bullet had entered behind his left ear, passed through the skull, lateral and inferior to the cerebellum, out the occiput and lodged in the posterior neck, partially shattering the atlas and axis. The patient was non-verbal and in a wheelchair. We were having a lot of trouble extracting an Energy Cyst from his head and neck. Then it occurred to me that we had to connect with the anger or insanity of the shooter to get release of the Energy Cyst.

I simply asked the shooter's emotion/energy to come out of the wound. I made this request aloud. There were several of us working during this session. We all felt the rage and insanity as the Energy Cyst slowly released through the mastoid process behind the left ear. I kept hearing in my mind the shooter screaming, "F____ you! F ____ you!" over and over.

This patient has gotten off his plateau since this session. His attitude was better. He showed signs of talking and regaining a little motor control and sensation in his legs.

2. The second experience was with two teenage girls who were riding in the same car when it was hit by another car. Following intuition, we put the two patients on parallel tables. I positioned myself between them, the driver was on my left and the passenger on my right.

Both had amnesia about much of the accident. We were able to re-experience the accident together and release the forces that went into the car in which they had been riding. As we did so, much anger, which had previously been denied, surfaced and we talked about the driver of the other car. One of these patients is wheelchair bound and the other has some third and fifth cranial nerve deficit that has been residual. It was a most effective session. We actually elicited a little sympathy for how the driver of the other car must feel. Previously, we had worked intensively on both patients and had been unable to re-experience the accident, unable to connect with repressed anger and certainly were unable to get them to consider how the driver of the other car must feel about the damage that resulted from the accident.

The girl in the wheelchair can now support her full weight on her right leg since the session described above. Both girls are now willing to meet and discuss the accident with the woman who hit them.

This is SomatoEmotional Release today.

Chapter III
Vector/Axis Integration
and Alignment

VECTOR/AXIS INTEGRATION AND ALIGNMENT

The technique that we have named "Vector/Axis Integration and Alignment" is something that I have been doing intuitively and largely in a nonconscious way for more than 15 years. I cannot tell you when it started because it was done without my realizing that I was doing it. Suffice it to say it began in the early 1970s.

It was during an Advanced CranioSacral Therapy seminar just a few years ago that one of the students, Adam, asked me what, exactly, I was doing. I evaded giving a precise answer. He repeated his question rather insistently. I realized that I was not aware of what I was doing nor why.

Whatever it was, it just happened as I allowed my hands and the rest of my body to do what felt appropriate for the patient. It was very subtle. It involved use of the extremities in movements of tractioning, torquing, side bending, compressing, waiting and so on. Most of the passive movements I did with the patient's body were very small. On occasion, however, I might move the ankles several inches to accomplish an effect in the torso. I always felt a sort of "falling into place" at the correct position. After this "falling into place" occurred, there was sense of stabilization or melding into position. This work was usually the finishing touch.

Adam continued his questioning and the rest of the group began to gather around. I was trying to formulate answers as I was standing at the supine patient's feet. Suddenly, I saw sparkling, very active, energetic lines superimposed within, not on, the patient's body. Structurally they resembled the stick people that most of us drew as children (and sometimes as adults). The lines were so shiny and energetic that they looked like the sparklers we use to help us celebrate the Fourth of July. The difference was (and still is) that the Fourth of July sparklers only sparkle in one place. These were sparkling lines in the patient's body. Since then, I frequently have seen these sparkling lines outside the patient's body in abnormal circumstances.

In this first instance, however, the sparkling lines all appeared to be within the patient's body. There was one line from the level of the upper border of the pubes straight up the center of the body to the head, with the exception that the line was interrupted just below the respiratory diaphragm. There were two horizontal sparkling lines. One ran from shoulder to shoulder and the other ran from hip to hip. These sparkling horizontal lines connected with the sparkling but infra-diaphragmatically interrupted, centrally-located, anatomically vertical line. At the lateral ends of both transverse lines were hinges that allowed the transverse lines to angulate with the positions of the four limbs. This allowed the sparkling lines to be longitudinally and centrally located in each arm from shoulder to hand and in each leg from hip to foot. In this patient (which was the first time I ever saw these sparkling lines) the hinge at the right shoulder seemed somehow disrupted. The right arm line was not connected to the shoulder-to-shoulder transverse line at its lateral end. The transverse line through the hips was at a 10-degree diagonal. The right end was superior and the left end was inferior, but the hinges were connected so that the sparkling lines in the legs were connected to the transverse line. Although the sparkling lines would have been consistent with unequal physical leg length, the physical legs were of equal length judging from the levels of malleoli.

I pointed out these sparkling lines to Adam and the rest of the group who had gathered around. Adam immediately asked what theses lines were because he could see them too. Without hesitation I heard myself say that the lines were "vectors." Vectors of what, I did not know. It did seem that these vectors were highly energetic. It also seemed that the disruptions at the infradiaphragmatic level and in the right shoulder hinge should somehow be connected. And that the transverse vector from hip to hip should be repositioned from a diagonal position to transverse symmetry.

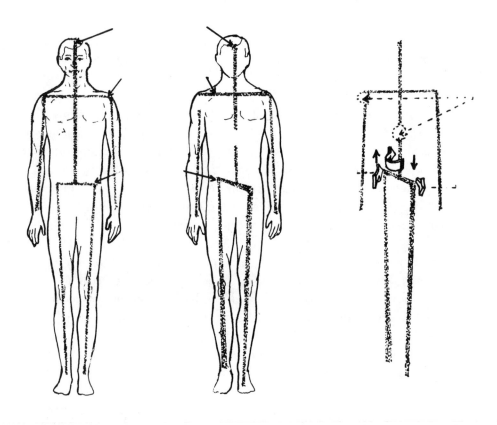

The two figures on the left compare the ideal Vector/Axis system with the system we first visualized. To the right, the Vector/Axis system is extracted from the body for clarification.
Illustration III – 1

As you might guess, the next question from the students was, "What do we do with those vectors?" I heard myself reply without hesitation that we simply put them together where the continuity is disrupted and we straighten, balance or reposition as indicated. At this point, I realized that this was what I had been doing nonconsciously and intuitively for so many years.

To demonstrate to the class how I would go about integrating and aligning this patient's vector system I had to allow my hands to have their way, doing what I had been doing intuitively for some time. It was a moment of truth. Was I being permitted to "see" what I had been working with all along or were these two separate systems I sensed—one with my hands and one with my eyes? Would the movements my hands did with the patient's body connect the disruptions in the vector system that I was seeing for the first time?

I thought how fortunate it was that the Advanced Class had only 10 people. One of them was the patient on the table. We were all good friends by now so I would not be making a fool of myself in front of a large, possibly antagonistic audience if this didn't work as I intuited that it would. I let my hands tell me what to do. We saw the vectors reconnect where they were disconnected. We could kinesthetically, as a group, sense when the separated ends came together and we could feel when they were securely melded into a single vector. It was not as obvious kinesthetically when the diagonal hip-to-hip vector moved but we could see it happening. When the position of balance was achieved, there was a sense of "falling into place." Most of the students felt this phenomenon occur. It was exciting to be able to "see" the effect of what I was doing. I shall now attempt to describe to you what I did.

First, I decided to balance/correct the relationship of the horizontal pelvic hip-to-hip vector with the vertical central vector. This decision was arbitrarily intuitive or vice versa. I am sure that I would have done just as well if I had integrated and aligned the right arm with the right shoulder first. I did horizontal-vertical vector alignment by simply tractioning the right leg and compressing the left leg simultaneously and very gently. The focus of attention was at the hips. I was using the legs as long levers to move them. My hand contact with the patient's body was at the feet. I was cradling one heel in each hand. I was lifting the feet and legs to the upper thigh area just slightly up and off the table to reduce bodily friction with the table top. As the vector appeared to align horizontally, I became aware that there was an abnormal rotation around a vertical axis. The right lateral end of the horizontal vector was posterior and the left lateral end was anterior. (I want to emphasize at this point that NONE of these vector misalignments had any correlation to physical body misalignment, but we can use the physical body to move the vectors if we go slowly and carefully. It is as though there is a magnetic attraction between the physical body and the vector when the system is energized adequately.) Anyhow, I rotated the pelvis a little in a counterclockwise direction from my vantage point at the feet until a very palpable "falling into place" sensation was felt—by me and the rest of the class who were NOT touching the patient. Once I felt this "falling into place," it seemed proper to wait a few seconds (perhaps 10 seconds) until the vector seemed to settle in and be "happy" in its realigned position. (I have found that if you move the body too soon after achieving the desired vector alignment, you can lose vector continuity or the vector will distort again as you replace the body parts in question.)

Next, I reattached the right arm vector to the shoulder. First, I straightened the arm until the arm vector was on a horizontal line with the transverse shoulder vector. Then I compressed the arm medially until I could see the two ends of the disconnected vectors come together. At this point, kinesthetic sense and intuition took over. I felt the two ends come together. They felt as though some sort of "hooking" was required, much as you might hook or rotate the arm of a mannequin into position to attach it. First, I rotated just about a 90-degree quarter turn counterclockwise (looking from lateral to medial), as though to line up the mecha-

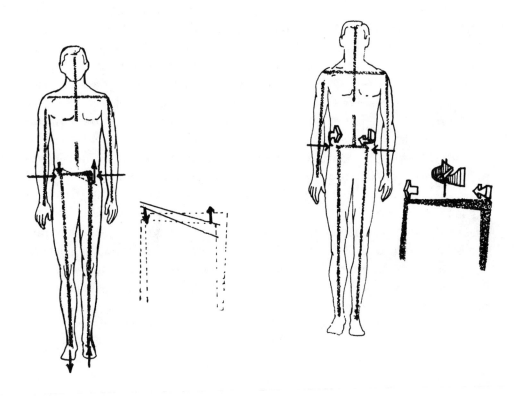

Shows how transverse hip-to-hip Vector/Axis was corrected in relationship to the vertical central Vector/Axis. See text.
Illustration III – 2

nism. Then I slowly rotated about 60 degrees clockwise until I felt the arm fall into place. The students also felt this falling into place sensation. Again I waited, perhaps 30 seconds this time, until the vector union seemed stable to me. This sensation of stability was like a sigh of relief as the two vectors melded together. (Oddly enough, everyone in the room with me seemed to know when the melding was complete, even though they were not touching the patient.)

Next, I placed one hand under the sacrum and the other hand under the lower thoracic spinal region. I compressed the lower spine into the thoracic region until I could see and feel the infradiaphragmatic vector disruption connect into continuity. We all felt it when the ends touched. We waited for a few seconds until it seemed stable, then took my hands away. Re-examination of this patient's vector system using the visualization of the shiny, sparkling lines revealed an integrated and highly energetic visible vector system imposed in the patient's body.

I must confess, this initial attempt to comprehend, visualize, explain and teach these little finishing touches was pretty astonishing to all of us. After this first demonstration, we had two full days of class remaining. We continued to experiment and play with the sparkling lines, the concepts and the techniques. It was a mind-blowing two days. Here we were, all pretty much seeing the previously invisible and feeling the previously "non-feelable." In view of these circumstances, it is most remarkable that we achieved a high level of agreement regarding that which we sensed. I'm not sure that I know what to make of this sudden piece of insight and the expansion and integration of my visual and kinesthetic abilities into a conscious level. I do know that it is a teachable technique. Since that first time, I have put this subject into the format of the SomatoEmotional Release workshop. In these circumstances, we teach about 40 students at a time to "see" the sparkling lines. Most of them can do it in one afternoon. I also know that the results are reproducible. (We should, I know, carry out a double-blind, controlled inter-examinator reliability study, but there just hasn't been time to think about that yet. The insights have been too exciting and moving so fast that to take time out to do a piece of reproducibility research right now seems beyond the realm of possibility.) I also know that patients/clients/subjects are very much aware of the positive effects of Vector/Axis Integration and Alignment when it has been done for them. Their remarks consistently relate to a sense of "improved connectedness" and "better body awareness" (proprioception).

I put in the word "axis" because vector implies motion or force. This is not always the case. I do not wish to imply that I believe that a force in a direction is always a component of these sparkling lines. On the other hand, there does seem to be a direction of energetic force in some people. Therefore, for the sake of clarity, I have begun using the combined term "Vector/Axis" for the visualized sparkling lines that we see superimposed in the patient. Many therapists see the lines with individualized characteristics. Some see them as blue lines, some as gold or yellow lines and so on. I can only tell you how I see them.

In a 1990 workshop that we were co-presenting, Marty Rossman, M.D., said that his experiences and observations would lead him to believe that when an individual is introduced to a new concept or therapeutic approach, the first experiences are the most miraculous. Then things settled down a little. One of my first experiences with the newly visualized Vector/Axis Integration and Alignment system fits Marty's statement perfectly. It was very soon after this technique came into my consciousness that a male lead dancer from a major ballet company was referred to

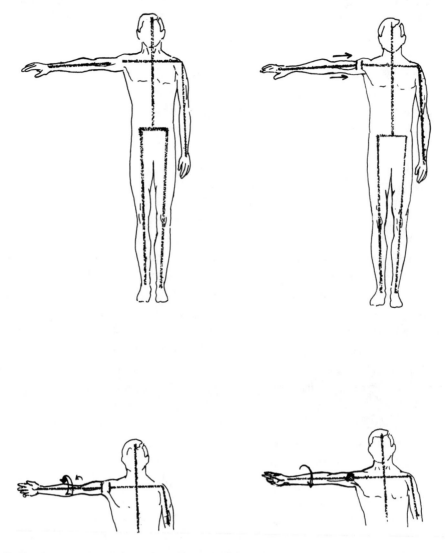

Steps to reconnect and align the Vector/Axis of the right arm with the lateral end of the shoulder-to-shoulder transverse Vector/Axis. See text.
Illustration III – 3

us for evaluation and treatment. He had been dancing with this ballet troupe for about six years and had been doing lead work most of that time when he was afflicted with a non-malignant tumor of the spinal cord. The tumor was in the mid-thoracic region at the level of the eighth thoracic spinal cord segment. Successful surgical excision had been accomplished about six months earlier. His surgical recovery was without incident or complication. He had begun physical therapy shortly after surgery.

At the time he presented at our facility, he was walking with a cane. His gait was stiff and tentative. He swung his legs laterally a bit as he walked. He stated that he was having a very difficult time making his legs do what he wanted them to do.

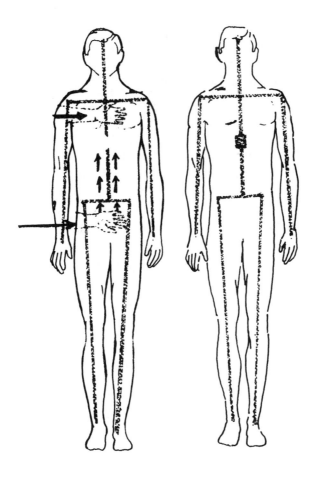

Method used to reconnect the infradiaphragmatic disruption
of the central Vector/Axis. See text.
Illustration III – 4

As a dancer, he was used to having his body do just what he asked of it. He was also used to knowing exactly where his body parts were. He had lost some of this knowledge of body position (without looking)—called proprioception. Naturally, his body performance and awareness expectations and requirements were much greater than those of the average person.

He came to us for two weeks of treatment. He had a total of eight appointments with me. My first and dominant finding was the lack of longitudinal mobility of the dural tube. It was very restricted in the middle and lower thoracic region. I feel fairly safe in saying that this restriction was most likely due to post-operative adhesion, membranous cohesion and unresolved tissue edema. I spent the first two and one-half to three sessions almost completely focused on dural tube mobilization. I worked it from both ends using the occipital and sacral handles. Some of our time had to be invested in the mobilization of these handles. I used multiple CV-4 techniques to force fluid down the dural tube. I performed V-spread techniques from anterior to posterior for the dural tube through the thorax as well as between the cranial crown and the sacrococcygeal complex in both superior-inferior and inferior-superior directions.

(It takes some time to direct energy the total length of the dural tube, but it is well worth the investment. Send the V-spread energy from one end toward the other and continue sending it until you feel its arrival in the receiving hand. If you're going to do it, do it. Take your time and make sure that you do it correctly and that you complete the task. You will feel the therapeutic pulsation, the heat and finally the sense of release in your receiving hand.)

With the dural tube mobilized, he noticed an immediate improvement in motor coordination. His legs obeyed commands that they had not obeyed for some time; his knees bent more readily and as he directed. By the end of the first week, his motor coordination was significantly improved in his opinion, but his proprioception improvements were not living up to his expectation. When he did a leap, he wasn't sure when his feet would touch the floor nor whether they were in the correct position.

I tried my new technique, Vector/Axis Integration and Alignment. This was about three weeks after my sight of the sparkling lines. I saw a very prominent disruption of his central vertical Vector/Axis. The gap between the two disconnected ends was about six inches long. It ran from mid-sternum down into the epigastrium. The task was to fill the gap, to meld the two ends of the disconnected Vector/Axis together. I tried pushing energy in from his head down, from his pelvis up and finally from his feet upwards. As I watched, I could see the sparkling energy building at the disconnected ends, but the ends did not get closer to each other. I decided to try to bring these ends together manually at the site of the disruption in the continuity of the central Vector/Axis.

This simplistic approach seemed a little "off the wall" at the time, even to me. But what was there to lose? I knew I couldn't hurt anything, so I tried. It took a couple of minutes before anything happened, then the disconnected ends began to move toward each other, closing the gap. In a short time, they abutted each other but the ends did not seem to meld together. I went back to the patient's head and gently pushed in a caudad direction, holding this push until I felt the now familiar falling into place sensation. This sensation was followed by a sense that the two ends were now melding together. Then there was a sense of relaxation, as though the resistance had gone. I then went to his feet and gently tractioned down. The central vertical Vector/Axis maintained its integrity. His Vector/Axis system seemed normal, intact and very "sparkly" to me. I asked him to try it out. He did not ask me what I had done, and I did not volunteer any explanation.

The next day he reported that for the first time since his tumor began to bother him he knew exactly where his feet were when he leaped into the air and returned to the floor. He knew precisely when they were about to strike the floor and he felt in total control of the position of his feet and legs as he landed. We both rejoiced and were astonished at how quickly his body awareness had returned after this session of Vector/Axis Integration and Alignment. It was as though it had never been gone. I spent the rest of his sessions exercising his craniosacral system, increasing his dural tube mobility and re-evaluating his Vector/Axis system. Actually, there was little left for me to do but I kept looking for more even though I didn't find it. His craniosacral system and Vector/Axis systems remained intact and in excellent working order.

In the fall of 1988, he returned to rehearsals with his ballet company. He had resigned himself to the idea that his career as a professional ballet performer was finished. He had decided to teach and to coach with his company. Now this crazy technique that we call Vector/Axis Integration and Alignment—coupled with the other crazy technique called Dural Tube Mobilization—had given him another chance at his career.

Since that first emergence of the Vector/Axis system into my conscious awareness, I have received several reports from others to whom we have presented this technique. The clinical results on a subjective and anecdotal level seem to be quite excellent. The techniques have been very rapidly assimilated into several therapists' armamentarium. The beauty of the concept seems to echo the whole of CranioSacral Therapy: it is a no-risk technique. It consumes minimal time, but the time must be one-on-one with the patient. It is an open-ended technique. Just as CranioSacral Therapy forces you to develop your perceptions, skills, attitudes and philosophies so that new vistas open for you, so does Vector/Axis Integration and Alignment. When you practice this technique, it develops and expands your sensory limits. An unknown universe awaits further exploration.

Now let us consider some clinical observations that I have made and that have been reported to me since we first added Vector/Axis Integration and Alignment to our curriculum. Sometimes the Vectors/Axes are outside the boundaries of the physical body. In such cases, I use the physical body much as I would a magnet to collect the Vector/Axis that is displaced. After the Vector/Axis settles into the body and stabilizes itself within the physical body, the body is used to manipulate the Vector/Axis into its correct position of alignment or to reconnect the separated end of a disrupted area.

You must allow time for the Vector/Axis to meld into the proper position in the physical body before you attempt to use the body as a vehicle to move the Vector/Axis. It is as though the body can be used as a time lapse magnet for the Vector/Axis. If you move the physical body too soon or too fast, you lose the Vec-

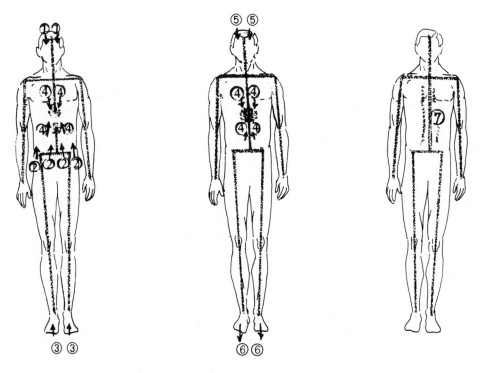

The steps used to reconnect the central vertical Vector/Axis after
surgical excision of a spinal cord tumor. See text.
1) Compression of head into trunk in attempt to approximate disrupted Vector/Axis ends
— unsuccessful.
2) Similar attempt at approximation from pelvis — unsuccessful.
3) Similar attempt at approximation from feet — unsuccessful.
4) Achieved approximation working locally at site of interruption of Vector/Axis continuity.
5) Compression of head into body is now helpful.
6) Traction at feet does not disconnect vertical Vector/Axis.
7) Integrity of Vector/Axis is maintained.
Illustration III – 5

tor/Axis. That is, you overcome the magnetic attraction between the physical body and the Vector/Axis. If you do lose it, no harm is done. Just go back, collect your Vector/Axis and try again.

Vector/Axis continuity is definitely disrupted or distorted by Energy Cysts, somatic dysfunctions, physical trauma, emotional disturbances and the like. If you integrate and realign the Vector/Axis system but do not resolve the underlying problem, the Vector/Axis will move back into its disrupted or misaligned pattern very quickly—occasionally I have seen this return to abnormality occur in a matter of seconds. This characteristic has an up side as well as a down side. On the up side, you can use the system to discover whether there is an underlying physical or emotional problem that has gone either undetected or unresolved and is causing the disruption or misalignment of the Vector/Axis system.

With some ingenuity, you can determine a great deal about the nature and significance of the underlying problem from the rapidity, location and severity of

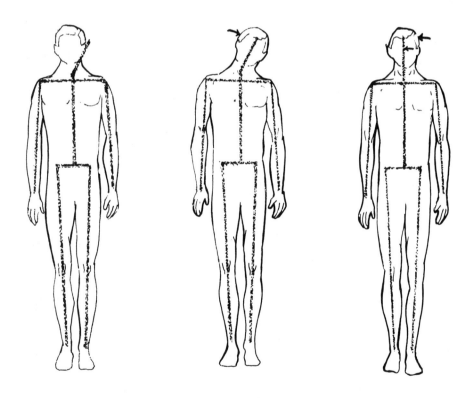

Use of the physical head and neck to "collect" and return to a normal position an energetic Vector/Axis that is displaced from the physical body. See text.
Illustration III – 6

the recurring Vector/Axis disruption or misalignment. You can tell about rejection of body parts that the patient considers to have committed offending acts or have not performed up to demand or expectation. There may be resistance to getting well. Or there may be missed Energy Cysts, missed somatic dysfunctions or other emotional reasons for the continuation of the repetitive disruption of the Vector/Axis system.

Once, when demonstrating before a SomatoEmotional Release class, I did a successful reconnection of a separated central vertical Vector/Axis. This separation was below the waist. The subject was a student volunteer. Within a few seconds of finishing the reconnection several student observers and I witnessed the reseparation of this central vertical Vector/Axis.

Again, I reconnected the Vector/Axis and it promptly reseparated. This reseparation occurred three times before I caught on. After the third reconnection and separation, the volunteer student patient went into a SomatoEmotional Release process that involved re-experiencing and releasing the effects of an unwanted pregnancy and abortion. She then completed a natural obstetrical delivery process as though the pregnancy had gone to completion. This process of completing the natural delivery process seems instinctive in humans. (It probably is instinctive in animals too, but this is beyond my experience.) She also confronted and resolved the hidden guilt about killing her baby through the abortion. She confronted and accepted her sexuality, though it was her sex drive that had gotten her into this predicament initially. In essence, she came face-to-face with her libido, the existence of which she had tried to deny since the pregnancy-abortion experience.

In her attempt to deny her sexuality and the existence and character of her libido, she had interrupted the continuity of her vertical central Vector/Axis between the waist and the pubes. Before we could get a lasting reconnection of this central Vector/Axis, she had to forgive herself and accept her sexuality as a natural part of her. With some dialogue and negotiation, she readmitted her pelvis and its organs to her total being. She forgave herself. The Vector/Axis was then reconnected and remained intact.

Since that experience, I have become aware of several cases of emotionally based body part rejection which manifested as Vector/Axis separations and misalignments. A very interesting example was that of a young man whose complaint was of right arm and shoulder pain. He could think of no particular incident or injury that might have caused the pain. He just woke up with it about eight months earlier. He had received several types of treatment, but the problem did not respond to any of them. It seemed to be getting progressively worse. It was not really an acute problem, but it was enough to prevent him from throwing a baseball or passing a football with his son. The patient had been a quarterback on his high school football team and wanted very much for his son, now 12 years old, to excel on the high school team in a few years.

We went through an Energy Cyst release that was mostly physical during the first visit. After this first session, I noted that the right arm vector was disconnected from the lateral end of its transverse shoulder Vector/Axis. Also, the right side of the transverse shoulder Vector/Axis was disconnected from the central vertical Vector/Axis. (See Illustration III - 7.)

I straightened the arm to horizontal and compressed medially, attempting to attach both separations simultaneously. I was successful and the reconnection lasted for three minutes. Then it went right back to the double separation again. On the next visit, SomatoEmotional Release revealed that he was rejecting his right arm because of a bad pass he had thrown in an "important" football game. The pass was

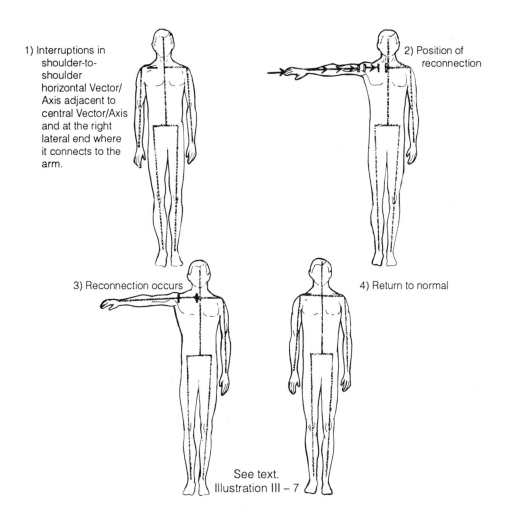

1) Interruptions in shoulder-to-shoulder horizontal Vector/Axis adjacent to central Vector/Axis and at the right lateral end where it connects to the arm.

2) Position of reconnection

3) Reconnection occurs

4) Return to normal

See text.
Illustration III – 7

intercepted and the game was lost. This was his last game as a high school football player. He did not attend college, so it was the end of his football career. He was really angry with his right arm and shoulder. They had performed badly at a very important time in his life. As his son's entry into high school status loomed closer and as he tried to teach his son to be a quarterback and pass a football, his rejected arm and shoulder became more and more symptomatic.

Through dialogue and negotiation with his arm and shoulder an amicable relationship was achieved. He forgave and accepted his arm and shoulder. I reconnected the Vector/Axis system where it was separated (as in Illustration III-7). This time, the reconnection held. His arm and shoulder function have returned to normal. (I hope his son doesn't take his football career as seriously as his father did.)

Recently, I became aware that an intuitive approach that I have been using with scoliosis patients also involves the Vector/Axis system. It has yet to be proven efficacious and that proof may never be forthcoming, but it seems right to me and I want to share the idea with you.

Before I get into the Vector/Axis system part, I should give you some background about how I view and treat scoliosis. First, I use arcing to search for specific active lesions along the torso. I am looking for the lesion that is key to the spinal curvature. The idea I have in mind relates to the possibility that the messages to large muscle groups regarding the level of idling contraction may be coming from small intervertebral or paravertebral muscles that are strained and signaling large muscle groups to over-contract. That is, the proprioceptors from small muscles could be sending incorrect information to the large muscles that are involved in maintaining postural stance.

(A few years back I had access to a thermography machine and I would scan the patient's body thermographically in addition to a very thorough arcing evaluation. As an aside, the two processes did, indeed, confirm one another in about 70 percent of the discovered hot lesions. As you might expect, arcing discovered deep active lesions that the thermography was cheated out of by the thickness of tissue interposed between the hot spot and the heat detectors. The agreement was very good in the paravertebral and rib cage areas, however.)

I search for these strained small muscles and attempt to relax them in my treatment of scoliotic patients. For a time, I injected these small muscles with a local anesthetic to test the hypothesis. Although temporary, there does seem to be a positive effect on spinal curvature after injection of specific paravertebral, intervertebral and intercostal hot spots.

I couple this approach with a balancing of the craniosacral system. My initial focus is on the dural tube and its bone attachments at the occiput, the second and third cervical vertebral bodies, the second sacral segment within the canal and on the coccyx. In addition, you must consider all the dural sleeves that attach at the intervertebral foramina. To get a balance without undue stress on the dural tube, it is of course necessary to evaluate and release any abnormal tensions in the total intracranial membrane system. This condition requires that the cranial vault, cranial base, hard palate, mandible and TMJs, the hyoid and its related muscles all be made functional.

Once you accomplish this, you must mobilize and balance the vertebral column, the pelvis and the extremities. (Now we get to the part that includes the Vector/Axis system.) Essentially I have removed, as best I can, all the factors that cause distortions and disruptions in this Vector/Axis system. At the end of each session I realign and integrate the Vector/Axis system. I use it as an index to reflect the ongoing presence of dysfunctions, Energy Cysts and emotions that may continue to disrupt its organization and integrity.

Besides this use of the Vector/Axis system, I have a strong feeling that if we can maintain the straightness of the central Vector/Axis and achieve spinal mobility at the same time, the straightness of the central Vector/Axis will influence (albeit slowly) the mobile spine toward straightness. Therefore it is important that the scoliotic patient/client be seen once or twice a week because keeping the central Vector/Axis as straight as possible for as much time during the week as possible is important.

I have consciously used this approach with only a few scoliotics since the idea hatched, so I cannot speak about it with the authority derived from vast clinical experience. Even had I been aware of the idea before, the question is: How can you assign the correct percentage of therapeutic effect to the Vector/Axis work when you are doing so many other therapeutic things concurrently? For those of you who wonder, yes I do evaluate leg length, but I don't assign it as high a priority as do many specialists in the area of spinal curvature or straightness. I do like to teach people what straightness feels like so that this perception of straightness can get into their nonconscious. I also investigate possible emotional reasons for spinal curvature. These emotional reasons, when present, may well cause recurrent distortions of the vertical central "sparkling line."

EXERCISES IN VECTOR/AXIS INTEGRATION AND ALIGNMENT

Now let's try some sample problems to illustrate how I would integrate and realign some distorted and disrupted Vector/Axis systems. We will need a set of symbols to use that can represent three-dimensional relationships and various dynamic processes. They are as follows:

SYMBOLS

1.   Disruption in continuity of the Vector/Axis in question.

2.   Vector/Axis is realigned but not melded together as yet. The ends are butted against each other.

3.   Vector/Axis is now melded together.

4.   Dot indicates pivot point. Line from dot to arrows is previous position of Vector/Axis with bend in it. Arrows indicate distance and direction of repositioning.

5.   Direction of force applied by therapist.

6.   Rotate part in one direction and then in the other in order to hook the two ends of the separated Vector/Axis together.

7.   Energy accumulates at point of disruption but separated ends do not approximate each other.

1) Vertical central Vector/Axis is interrupted and bent.
2) Transverse hip-to-hip Vector/Axis is misaligned in relation to vertical central Vector/Axis.
3) Right leg Vector/Axis extends inferior to the foot of the physical body.

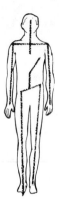

Illustration III – 8

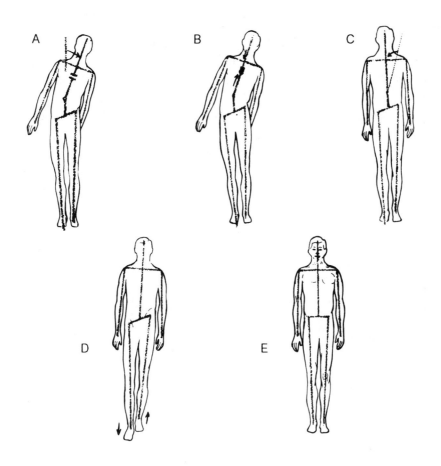

Correction of the Vector/Axis system using Option 1, Sample problem 1
as described in text.
Illustration III – 9

Sample Problem 1

Suppose you visualize a Vector/Axis system superimposed in the body that looks like Illustration III-8. What would you do?

As I see it, there are two choices in the initial approach. First, you could attempt to correct the vertical central Vector/Axis from above. The advantage is that it gives you an integrated and aligned central vertical Vector/Axis with which to align the hip-to-hip transverse Vector/Axis. The realignment of the lower transverse Vector/Axis is then more easily carried out.

Let's look at the steps we must take to integrate and realign the Vector/Axis system if we use the first alternative:

Move the entire lower part of the physical body until the bend in lower vector is straightened, as in Figure A. At the same time, push the right leg up and pull the left leg down to get the right angle position of hip-to-hip Vector/Axis in relationship to the lower half of the vertical central/vector, as in Figure B, Illustration III – 9. During this later process you will need to traction the right leg and compress the left leg first to get the Vector/Axis properly positioned in the physical body, as in Figure A. Then reverse the traction and compression forces to move the vector system once it has melded into its new position in the physical body, as in Figure B.

Reposition the lower physical body taking the Vector/Axis system with the body. Use the crossings of the midline by the central vertical Vector/Axis as the pivot point so that abutment of the separated ends of the central vertical Vector/Axis is obtained, as in Figure C. Wait for melding to occur, as in Figure D.

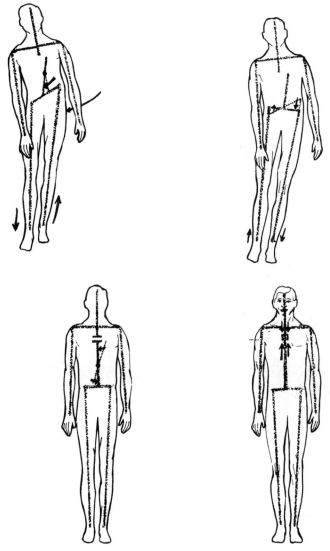

Correction of Vector/Axis system using option 2 as described on Sample Problem 1.
Illustration III – 10

The second alternative would be to correct the hip-to-hip transverse Vector/Axis and to straighten the bend in the lower vertical central Vector/Axis at the same time. Then connect the break in the mid-portion of the vertical central Vector/Axis as the second part of the maneuver.

I really don't have a preference about which option is best. It is a little more complicated if you use the second option because it forces you to do two things at once but it is also a little more fun. If you miss the first time, try again. There is no harm done and it seems that you have an almost infinite number of chances to succeed.

Sample Problem 2
This looks like a simple problem (Illustration III-11), and it is. But there is one little trick that goes with it that makes the treatment effective. Once you get the

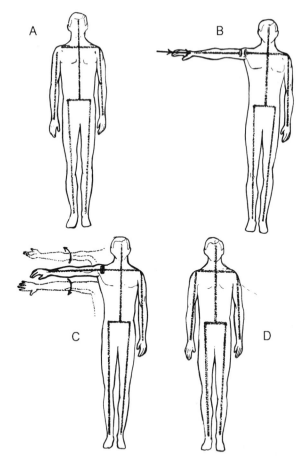

Correction for separation of the Vector/Axis system at the right shoulder. See text.
Illustration III – 11

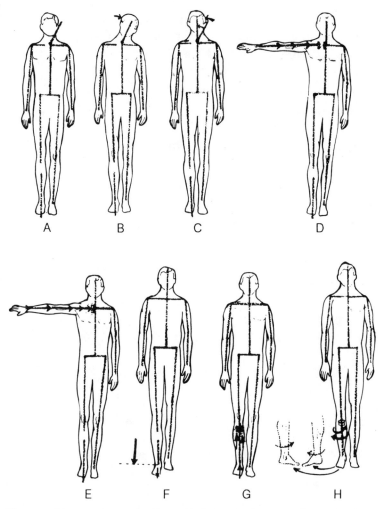

Three problems that require Vector/Axis integration and alignment. See text.
Illustration III – 12

arm and shoulder lined up, you have to screw it in just as you do the limb on a mannequin. Remember, the shoulders and hips are hinged so you may have to play around a little to find the proper abutment position.

Sample Problem 3

Here (Illustration III-12) we have three problems that require Vector/Axis integration and realignment. First, we have a central vertical Vector/Axis that is sharply bent to the left just above the junction with the shoulder-to-shoulder transverse Vector/Axis. Second, the shoulder-to-shoulder transverse Vector/Axis is interrupted just to the right of the central vertical Vector/Axis. Third, the right leg vector is separated at the knee and protrudes beyond the foot out of the physical body. See Figure A.

I would begin with the central vertical Vector/Axis because it is the foundation onto which we will attach the separated right shoulder-arm Vector/Axis. First, take the physical head-neck complex to the left. Be careful to bend the physical body abruptly at the sharp bend in the Vector/Axis. I suggest that you place one finger directly beneath the angle of this sharp bend. The pivot point must be precisely located. Wait until the Vector/Axis has settled into the physical head neck complex, as seen in Figure B.

When you sense that the settling-in process has been completed, carefully and slowly (while observing the Vector/Axis for slippage or disruption) return the physical head-neck complex to the neutral position. When the Vector/Axis is correctly positioned you will sense the falling into place. Wait for the settling process to complete. See Figure C.

Next, we will reconnect the right shoulder transverse Vector/Axis to the vertical central Vector/Axis and its counterpart on the left side. Position the arm horizontally and push in so that the correct position of abutment occurs. You may have to move the arm-shoulder complex anterior or posterior a little to obtain the correct position for abutment. Remember you are working in a three-dimensional system. See Figure D.

After you have found the correct position of abutment, wait for the melding process to complete, as in Figure E, then reposition the arm to the patient's side slowly and gently as in Figure F.

Next, we work with the right knee Vector/Axis separation. First, pull the physical leg inferiorly to reset the displaced distal segment of the Vector/Axis properly in place in the physical body, as seen in Figure F. Now compress the leg to cause abutment. Await melding as in Figure G. Rotation of the lower leg may be necessary to obtain proper Vector/Axis melding. See Figure H.

Sample Problem 4

This patient (Illustration III-13) presents us with a problem involving the central vertical Vector/Axis and the shoulder-to-shoulder horizontal axis. The central vertical Vector/Axis is disconnected just below its junction with the shoulder-to-shoulder Vector/Axis. The superior portion of the central vertical Vector/Axis is rotated in a clockwise direction when viewed from the front. The pivot point where the diagonal Vector/Axis crosses the midline is in the lower cervical region. The lower end of the diagonally displaced Vector/Axis has taken the horizontal shoulder-to-shoulder Vector/Axis with it to the patient's right. (See Figure A.)

To correct this problem, you must glide the transverse shoulder-to-shoulder Vector/Axis with the de-rotation of the central vertical Vector/Axis. As you take the clockwise rotation out of the central vertical Vector/Axis, you must maintain the lower cervical pivot point. Place one finger on the lower cervical spine at the pivot point. Move the head-neck physical complex around this pivot point to collect the central vertical Vector/Axis. Wait for settling in to occur. Also move both shoulders and arms so that you are collecting the vector system for those parts of the physical body. (See Figure B.)

Now use the physical head-neck complex to move the vertical central Vector/Axis in a counterclockwise rotation. At the same time, move the arms and shoulders to take the horizontal shoulder-to-shoulder and arm Vector/Axis to normal position. Obtain correct vertical position and abutment with the lower vertical central Vector/Axis as in Figure C. Wait for melding to complete between the previously disconnected ends. You may have to do some exploratory rotation of the head-neck complex around a longitudinal axis in order to achieve a proper result. (See Illustration III-13, Figure D.)

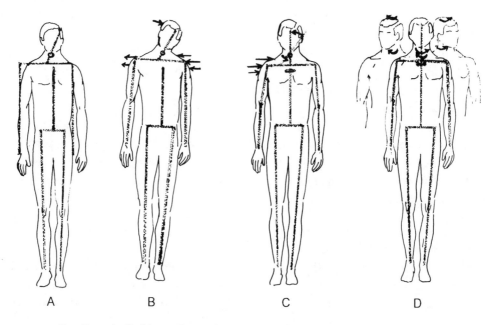

A   B   C   D

See Sample Problem 4 in text for description of problem and solution.
Illustration III – 13

Sample Problem 5

In this patient (Illustration III-14), we see a displacement of the shoulder-to-shoulder horizontal Vector/Axis to the right. All other Vector/Axes appear to be correctly integrated and aligned. See Figure A.

This problem is solved by slowly and gently moving the body with shoulder-to-shoulder Vector/Axis and the related arm Vector/Axis to the patient's left until the Vector/Axis line up, then move the body back to neutral. You may use the physical body, or you may simply move the energy lines. Either one will work. Be sure to watch the effect of what you do so you don't disrupt or bend the central Vector/Axis as you move the horizontal one. The same techniques can be used to correct a displaced hip-to-hip horizontal Vector/Axis.

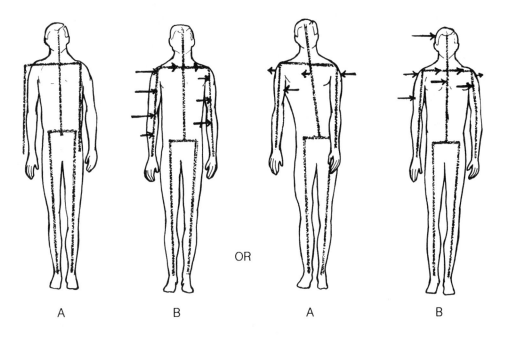

See Sample Problem 5 in text for description of problem and solutions.
Illustration III – 14

Sample Problem 6

In this patient (Illustration III-15), we see a central vertical Vector/Axis that has disconnected ends that are overriding. Besides lateral displacement, anterior/posterior displacement of the disconnected ends is frequently seen in this type of problem. There also may be a rotational displacement component between the two ends. You will have to watch closely and palpate delicately to determine what needs to be done. See Figure A, Illustration III-15.

This correction can be made by tractioning either the lower or the upper body so that the override of the two ends of the disconnected vertical central Vector/Axis is compensated. In Figure B you see a cephalad traction on the upper part of the body. To accomplish this traction, position both hands under the supine patient, palms up, with the patient's head resting on your forearms to guide the whole upper body effectively. Then move the Vector/Axis system using the physical body.

Next, move the whole upper body to the patient's left being sure to take the whole upper body Vector/Axis system with the physical body. You should be able to sense whether there is anterior/posterior or rotational displacement. If they are present, correct them with physical body movement while holding your traction. Search for abutment. (See Figure C.)

Wait for melding to occur. If it does not happen, you have missed a subtle anterior/posterior or rotational displacement. You may have to experiment a bit and see what feels right. I find it more difficult to visualize these subtle anterior/ posterior or rotational misalignments, so I depend more upon intuition and the feel of things.

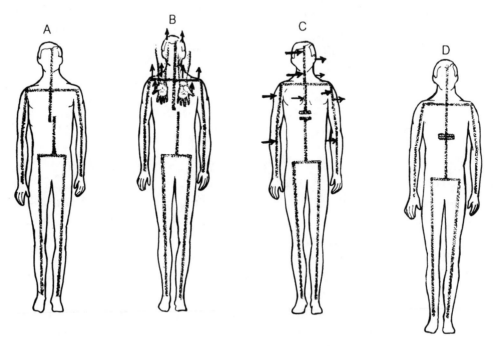

See Sample Problem 6 in text for description of problem and solution.
Illustration III – 15

The sample problems on the previous pages are intended to introduce some of the more common Vector/Axis system disconnections and misalignments that I have seen. There are many possible Vector/Axis system distortions. Each patient/client has patterns. Don't try to fit the individual patient/client into a preconceived pattern. Treat each patient/client as though there is something new and different about him or her. Your goal is to understand the pattern of each individual.

In these illustrated solutions, I have attempted to display the use of common sense in the correction of Vector/Axis system disruptions and misalignments. There are only a few simple rules that I have seen to be somewhat pervasive throughout the work:

- Emotional resistance can disrupt a Vector/Axis system almost as quickly as you integrate it, or it can prevent you from achieving even temporary integration.
- The physical body can be used as a magnet to move the energetic Vector/Axis system components.
- Where proper alignment or abutment occurs you feel it. So do others who may not be touching the body in question but are in the vicinity.
- Wait for settling in and melding to occur. You will feel this too. Once you have felt this sensation you will always remember it. So, it is much easier to learn this method of therapy in the presence of one who is experienced in the work who can guide you one on one.

Enjoy. This is a really fun game to play and yields truly amazing therapeutic results.

Chapter IV
Mouth, Face and Throat Work
Expanded and Revised

HARD PALATE PROTOCOL REVIEW

Time has passed, experience has accumulated and comprehension has increased. We now have greater appreciation of the total body release effects related to specific osseous, soft tissue and energy work that can be done on the mouth, face and throat.

1. In *CranioSacral Therapy (Volume I)* the focus is mostly on the osseous structures of the hard palate and on the releasing and balancing of the temporal bones and the mandible.
2. The book describes some work that deals with the temporalis, masseter and pterygoid muscles.
3. In *CranioSacral Therapy II, Beyond the Dura* we broaden the focus to include much more information about the whole masticatory system—its soft tissues and its relationships to the nervous system.
4. In this volume, I shall further describe how this region of the body interrelates with Energy Cyst release, SomatoEmotional Release, therapeutic imagery and dialogue.

Before beginning the in-depth mouth, face and throat work, it is necessary that you effectively carry out all the techniques of the 10-Step Protocol for the craniosacral system. There should be a special focus on the thoracic inlet, the occipital cranial base, the temporal bones and the whole intracranial membrane system. You should also complete preliminary balancing of the mandible. You may not have gotten total release of those parts of the system but you should have gotten at least partial release and be aware of the location and (I hope) the sources of any remaining restrictions.

After completion of the 10-Step Protocol, I suggest that you do the hard palate techniques in the order in which they are given in the CSTII workshop. The CSTII study guide also describes the techniques, so I will just review them in brief here.

Begin with evaluation of bilateral maxillary motion into the flexion and extension phases of the craniosacral motion. Remember, the hard palate widens during craniosacral flexion and narrows during extension. Evaluate for synchrony with the sphenoid, for symmetry of range of motion and for ease of motion. You will usually find some asymmetry and restriction. You can usually work through the transient dysfunctions by simply supporting the motion of the maxillae and coordinating it with the sphenoid motion.

If there is a non-transient restriction on one side or the other of the maxillae, you should initially do an indirect away-from-the-barrier releasing technique. Then go directly against the resistance if necessary. Get what you can with this technique. Be patient. I think you will not achieve full symmetry and synchrony until you have completed the remainder of the hard palate techniques.

Next evaluate for maxillary torsion to the left and to the right. Remember that maxillary hard palate torsion is non-physiologic motion. You are evaluating the hard palate's ability to accept and comply with this non-physiologic movement that you are inducing. Keep in mind that since you are torsioning the whole hard palate in this test you must stabilize the sphenoid against the abnormal motion you are putting into the system. If you do not stabilize the sphenoid you may well induce a dysfunctional motion pattern of the cranial base. Since the hard palate torsion is around the vertical axis the sphenoid would most likely be put into one of its vertical axis dysfunction patterns. This could be either side bending or lateral strain depending on how the occiput responds.

You also must keep in mind that it may require 10 or 20 seconds for the hard palate to respond around your torsional urging. DO NOT use more force because you have to wait. Just wait, please. Use, perhaps, up to 15 grams (three nickels) of force. DO NOT be guilty of inducing a hard palate dysfunction because you are impatient. As the hard palate complies with your torsional urging (around a verti-

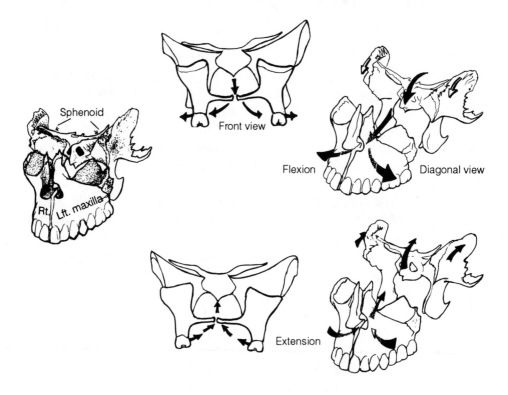

Direction of maxillary movement during the flexion and extension phases
of the craniosacral system.
Illustration IV-1

cal axis) to the left and to the right (or vice versa), compare the range and ease of motion of one direction with the other. If there is an asymmetry, do the corrections first indirectly and then directly against the resistance if the asymmetry persists.

The same rules apply to hard palate corrections on the cranial vault. Namely, use a small force for a longer time. You will not get an unwanted dysfunction. If you become impatient or too forceful, you are asking for trouble. Feel for the threshold in which the patient's body subtly begins to contract and protect itself against your intrusion. DO NOT work at a level of force that induces patient defense activity. BACK OFF and work at a level of energy that does not cause patient defenses to activate. If a torsion pattern does not seem correctable using the torsion techniques as described, it may be that you are dealing with a unilateral impaction between the sphenoid's pterygoid process and the palatino-maxillary complex on that side. You can usually tell if this is the situation when the sphenoid wants to follow the hard palate anteriorly and will not separate from the palatino-maxillary complex during the test for torsion. If you do find the spheno-palatino-maxillary

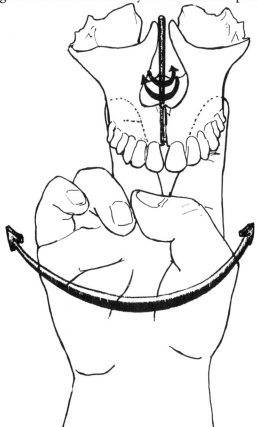

Finger positions in the mouth are shown. Arrows indicate the direction of force applied to the maxillae (through the teeth) to test for right and left torsion.
Illustration IV-2

complex moving as an inseparable unit, be patient. Exercise the joint. Perform torsion testing several times. If it still won't release, wait until you do the spheno-palatino-maxillary decompression work. Just remember that the impaction is present.

Next, we will evaluate for hard palate shear in relationship to the sphenoid. Shear is the descriptor we use for the evaluation technique that moves the hard palate transversely in relationship to the sphenoid. Again, you are inducing a non-physiologic motion so you must stabilize the sphenoid. By stabilizing, I simply mean not allowing the sphenoid to go with the hard palate. Wait for the response to occur first to one side and then to the other. DO NOT use more than 15 grams

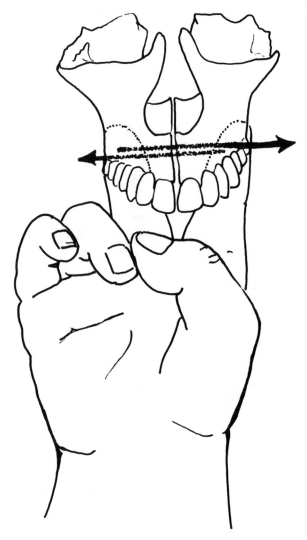

Finger placement and direction of force for hard palate shear to both right and left.
Illustration IV-3

(three nickels) worth of force. Be patient. Evaluate range and ease of motion for symmetry. If you find an asymmetry use the indirect technique first, then follow by going directly against the resistance. If you are successful in obtaining the release, celebrate. If you are not successful, be patient. Repeat the evaluation and treatment process a few times and go on to the next technique.

Next, we will decompress the hard palate from the sphenoid. To do this technique, we must again stabilize the sphenoid with one hand while we move the hard palate anterior with the other hand. For the supine patient, anterior is toward the ceiling. This technique will usually correct the residue of hard palate restrictions from torsion and shear. If there continues to be a unilateral compression (impac-

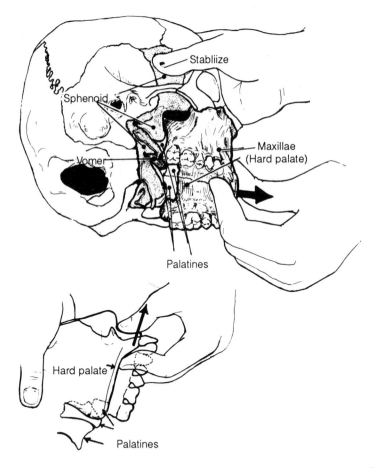

Direction of hard palate (maxillary) decompression technique is shown above. Finger position may vary. Sometimes, it is helpful to make finger contact with the biting surfaces of the posterior molars as you decompress. The proximity to the spheno-palatino-maxillary complex may be helpful. This is the same finger placement previously described for maxillary evaluation techniques.
Illustration IV-4

tion) between the hard palate and the sphenoid's pterygoid process, it means two things: One is that you must be patient and continue the hard palate anteriorly directed traction for a long time. Second, you probably have one helluva palatine problem.

After you feel that you have achieved decompression release as signified by independent anterior movement of the hard palate in relationship to the sphenoid, go back through the flexion, extension, torsion and shear evaluations and be sure. If you continue to find dysfunction, you may find it useful to do a V-spread at this juncture. If you still don't get perfect maxillary response, don't become obsessed. The maxillary may have done all that it can for the time being. Go on to the vomer and palatines. But before moving on, I should like to clarify a few points.

1.   The hand position for all the maxillary techniques is either with the index and middle fingers or the middle and ring fingers on the biting surfaces of the upper canine, premolar and molars. If the teeth are gone, take out the denture and apply your fingers directly to the gums. If the gums are slippery, wrap a little gauze around the fingers you are using. Ideally, your other hand should be in contact with the two great wings of the sphenoid. I can span most heads with my thumb and third or fourth finger. If you can get a thumb on one great sphenoid wing and a finger on the other great sphenoid wing, this is great. But there are lots of you who just don't have the size hand that can do that. If you cannot, apply your hand to the frontal bone. This bone does pretty much what the sphenoid does, so you can use it to stabilize the sphenoid and read what the sphenoid is doing through the frontal. If there are two therapists/facilitators working together, one of you can do the vault hold and work with the sphenoid while the other does the hard palate.

2.   Stabilizing the sphenoid can mean one of two things. You may stabilize it within its flexion-extension motion pattern. That is, you can support the movement and not let what you are doing with the maxillae interfere. Or you can stabilize the sphenoid in neutral and just hold it there. Prevent it from moving. Either method is acceptable.

3.   By indirect correction, we mean taking the tissue in question in the direction that it wants to go and holding it there. Here, we are talking about the maxillae (hard palate). For example, if the hard palate will torsion to the right more easily than it will torsion to the left, we take it to the right as far as it will go. We then hold it in that extreme right torsional position for several seconds (seldom more than half a minute). Don't use any more energy than necessary; just barely maintain the position. Usually after a few seconds the hard palate will move further into right torsion. This is the indirect release. The sphenoid will also feel as though something has released in it when this occurs. After this indirect release has occurred, follow the hard palate back to neutral and go into left torsion. Chances are, the hard palate will go further to the left than it did before. Follow it as far to the left as it will go. You will ultimately encounter resistance. Gently stay against this

resistance until a release occurs. This is the direct correction. After the direct release has occurred, move the hard palate gently as far as it will go to the left, then bring it back to neutral.

Wait a few seconds and re-evaluate to the right and to the left. You should find at least 50 percent improvement. If you don't, repeat the indirect-direct correction process or move on to the next step in the hard palate work and come back later to re-evaluate this restriction.

4.   I have selected the order of hard palate, (maxillary, vomer and palatine) evaluation and correction in this way because each step facilitates the next—that is flexion-extension release facilitates torsion correction. Torsion correction seems to ease shear correction, and all three of the aforementioned seem to help spheno-palatino-maxillary decompression (sphenoid-hard palate decompression).

5.   Non-physiologic motions that we induce for purposes of evaluation and correction should be induced during the neutral zone of craniosacral system activity. This timing seems to offer the least insult to this very sensitive system.

Now let us briefly review the vomer and palatine work that should be completed before moving on into the soft tissue and energy techniques involving the mouth, face and throat. The vomer is only indirectly but very effectively accessed through the roof of the mouth.

1.   Place the palmar surface of your finger on the midline of the roof of the patient's mouth and reach as far back as you can without activating the gag reflex. After you find this position with the pad of the distal end of your finger, position the rest of the palmar surface of your finger so that you get as much contact as you can get with the midline surface of the hard palate and the back of the middle incisor teeth.

2.   Now intention very strongly that you have a connection between your finger and the patient's vomer. As you know by now, intentioning works very well. You can evaluate vomer function and correct vomer dysfunction even though the maxillary bones are interposed between your finger and the vomer.

3.   Use your other hand to monitor the sphenoid or frontal, depending on your hand size. I still like to touch the thumb of my vomer hand to some part of my sphenoid (frontal) hand so that I have a good sense of the movements of the vomer and the sphenoid in relationship to each other. If I don't have contact between my two hands I can feel a little lost at times.

4.   First we evaluate vomer-sphenoid flexion-extension synchrony. As the posterior vomer comes inferiorly and the anterior vomer moves superiorly, the sphenoid should go into flexion. If this is not so, the vomer is out of synchrony with the sphenoid. To correct this situation, simply guide the vomer into synchrony with the sphenoid while you reinforce sphenoidal motion. Usually, I just hold the vomer still until the sphenoid catches up and then help the vomer move with the sphenoid. Most of the time this is easily done. The vomer is such a delicate bone; it

offers little resistance. When there is significant resistance to flexion-extension synchrony correction, it is usually because there is a severe vomer-sphenoid impaction. If this is the case, it will feel as though the vomer is a spoke protruding from the sphenoid body. In this situation, the vomer may not correct easily. Keep it in mind until you get to the vomer-sphenoid decompression technique (disimpaction).

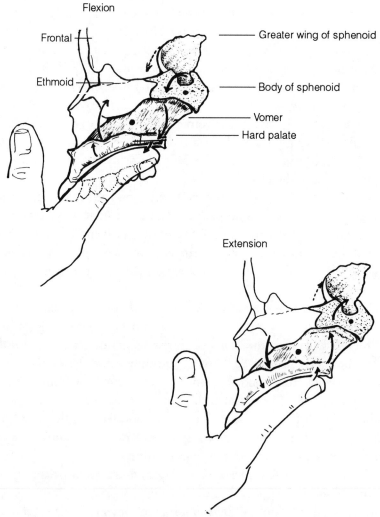

The above finger placement in the mouth is used for all vomer evaluation and treatment techniques with one exception (described under the sphenoid-vomer impaction treatment). The arrows indicate the direction of the motion of the vomer and the sphenoid during the flexion and extension phases of craniosacral motion.

Illustration IV–5

Don't worry. You'll come back to it. When you go through the torsion and shear evaluation and corrective techniques you will ease the disimpaction.

5.   To evaluate torsion of the vomer, it is preferable to support sphenoid motion because the constant movement helps to mobilize the vomer. If you don't feel comfortable supporting sphenoid motion, hold it immobile in neutral, but this is second best. Now torsion the vomer about a vertical axis envisioned through the cruciform suture which is about two-thirds of the way back from the front of the hard palate on the midline. Induce torsion both left and right. Compare range and ease of motion. Remember, the vomer is very delicate. You have to be alert and sensitive to detect restrictions to either torsion or shear in the vomer. You can easily correct it when you do find a torsion or a shear problem by just going through the evaluative process a few

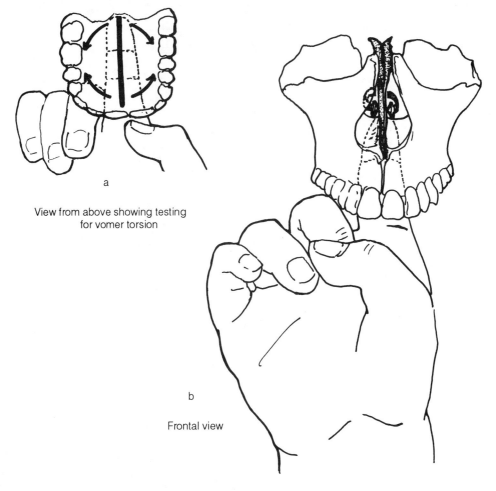

a

View from above showing testing
for vomer torsion

b

Frontal view

Finger placement and direction of torsion-inducing force directed at the vomer: right torsion (a) and left torsion (b). Note the pivot point.
Illustration IV–6

times. Occasionally, you may find it necessary to apply the indirect-direct corrective techniques described, but this will occur in a minority of cases.

6.   The evaluation of the vomer shear uses the same finger in the mouth position as the torsion techniques. But now we move straight lateral in one direction and then the other while either supporting the sphenoid in its motion pattern or holding it still in neutral. Compare the range and ease of motion for symmetry. When you find a dysfunction, go through the evaluation process a few times. This will usually correct it. If this doesn't work, use the indirect-direct technique I have previously described.

The difficult vomer problems are usually those of impaction between the sphenoid and the vomer. Remember, the sphenoid projects about one-quarter inch of bony lamina into the groove of the vomer. This projection is oriented in an anterior-inferior direction. Impaction of these two bones is usually due to trauma. Release of the impaction may require a great deal of patience on your part.

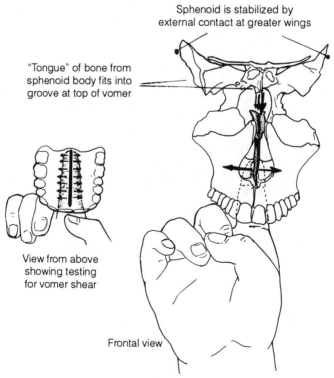

Finger position and direction of shear-inducing evaluation forces for the vomer.
Illustration IV–7

To evaluate the vomer for impaction with the sphenoid, we use the same finger on the hard palate midline position. I place my thumb either on the external surface of the gum over the maxillae on the midline, on the skin just between the nose and the lip on the midline or over the glabella. Use the position with which you feel most comfortable. The other hand *must* monitor the sphenoid (frontal). Then I apply a traction to the vomer in an anterior and slightly inferior direction. Now you must evaluate the sphenoid to see if it tenaciously follows the vomer or if there is only a little following tendency of the sphenoid when you induce vomer trac-

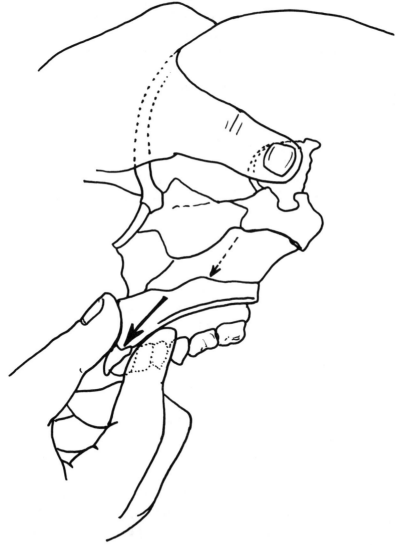

Hand position and direction of therapeutic force used to disimpact the vomer from the sphenoid. The thumb may be placed externally just below the nose or over the glabella.
Illustration IV–8

tion. (Normally, this tendency dissipates in 20 or 30 seconds.) After the sphenoid stops following the vomer, you can feel the vomer and sphenoid doing their hinging activity with flexion and extension of the craniosacral system and you can feel the vomer moving in the direction of your traction without dragging the sphenoid with it.

When significant impaction between vomer and sphenoid is present, the traction on the vomer will first interfere with normal sphenoid flexion-extension activity. Then as traction continues, it will tend to lift the sphenoid anteriorly, usually into an exaggerated position of extension. When this occurs, continue your vomer traction. Simultaneously try to encourage or induce normal flexion-extension activity of the sphenoid. You are trying to loosen the tongue of the sphenoid bone that is impacted within the invagination of the vomer, and you are trying to convince the maintaining connective tissues to relax. Work easily and gently. Be very patient. It is rather like pulling a large weed from your garden while trying to keep the root intact.

When the decompression or disimpaction between vomer and sphenoid occurs, the sphenoid will settle back posteriorly and the vomer will float up anteriorly in response to your traction. When this occurs, there is a wonderful sense of release that goes with it. Sometimes it is necessary to V-spread from the posterior occipital protuberance of the skull anteriorly to the "V" that you form by placing a finger on either side of the glabella and nose. You may also V-spread from inside the roof of the mouth through the top of the head to help loosen the impaction. Keep working; be patient; it will disimpact eventually. This can be a test of your patience and trust.

The palatines are next on your agenda. The hard palate has been loosened from the pterygoid processes as the maxillae were decompressed. We have done everything that we can do indirectly from the hard palate to release palatine bone dysfunction. Now you should evaluate the palatine directly. Very gently place a finger tip on the palatine bone as it presents itself in the roof of the mouth. It is medial to the posterior molars about one-quarter inch. The palatines, of course, divide on the midline of the hard palate so there are two of them, one on the left and one on the right. I always evaluate them separately. I have heard people say that they do both palatines at once. My fingers are too large to do that, so I cannot speak from personal experience. My bias is to do one at a time.

I place one finger on the palatine and the other hand over the top of the head like a skull cap. I like to feel the energy from my finger on the palatine come through to the receiving hand on the top of the head. Since the palatine has a vertical component that goes up and contributes to the floor of the orbit of the eye, I visualize this direction of energy as helping to release the upper part of the palatine bone. Once I feel the energy come through the top of the head, I physically elevate the palatine very gently as far as it will go. Then I move it laterally as far as it will go. Then I follow it medially and then inferiorly back to the neutral position. Repeat the process as often as you need on both sides. If there is residual compression between the hard palate and the pterygoid process of the sphenoid, of course the palatine will not respond normally to your test motions. If this is the case, you may have to return to the maxillary-sphenoid decompression technique to get the palatine freed up.

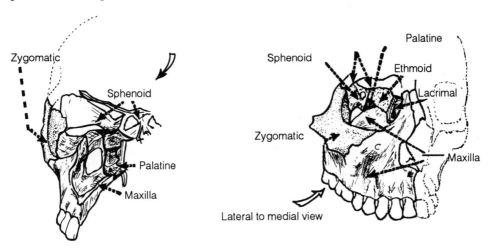

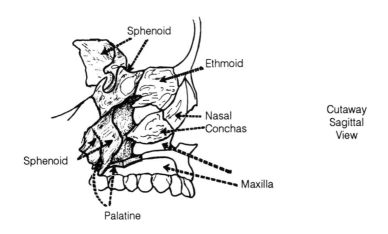

Finger placement for palatine evaluation and treatment techniques. Three views of the anatomy of the palatine bone and its related structures clearly demonstrate how palatine dysfunction can result in orbital symptoms.
Illustration IV–9a

It is not uncommon for a palatine bone to be restricted in a position that is cephalad to that which the bone would prefer. In these cases, the palatine will descend further than it elevates after release. Sometimes the palatine just doesn't want to elevate. Use GENTLE pressure of five grams or less over a long period. (Dick MacDonald hung out on my right palatine bone for 12 minutes once before it would move into elevation, so be patient.) Sometimes a palatine will go up and down but it won't move laterally. Here, go up with it as far as it will go and GENTLY hold it there with some lateral intention and urging as long as it takes. This may mean more than one session.

The most difficult palatine I ever encountered belongs to a very pleasant 28-year old lady. She'd had four wisdom teeth extracted a few years ago under general anesthesia. She had not been able to work or be comfortable since. There was a reactive scoliosis, a spasmodic torticallis, pelvic pain with dysmenorrhea, sternal pain and costochondritis, headache, neck pain, visceral disturbances and general

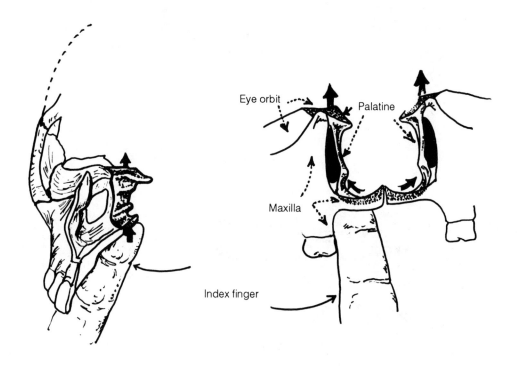

Finger placement for palatine evaluation and treatment techniques. Note how the superior movement of the palatine bone broadcasts to the eye.
Illustration IV–9b

depression. All this had occurred within a week of the dental extractions. I was doctor/therapist number 42 in her history! She claimed good health and function before the wisdom teeth extractions.

To make a long story short, after wading through the layers upon layers of reactions, adaptations and so on, they all pointed to her left palatine bone. (I have not yet been able to get total correction but when I get the palatine partially re-leased, all the symptoms abate temporarily.) The palatine was locked in a very superior position and it was most difficult to bring down. The maxilla on the same side was very much internally rotated. That too was most difficult to release. The zygoma seemed to offer the key. In the floor of the orbit of the eye, the orbital process of the palatine lay medial to the orbital part of the maxilla, which in turn lay medial to the orbital portion of the zygoma. The picture that I have is that during the forceful dental extraction, the left palatine was pushed cephalad so that the orbital process went up from its normal position. The palatine had become trapped in this cephalad position by the internal rotation and cephalad jamming of the maxilla on that side. Somehow the zygoma on that side was also jammed medi-ally. The zygoma maintained the malposition of the maxilla. The ethmoid fur-nishes much of the medial wall of the orbit. This bone contacts the maxilla and palatine which also had been forced into dysfunction.

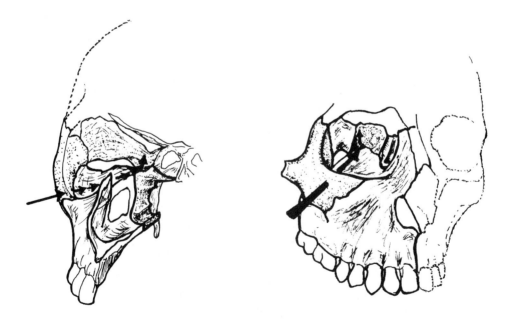

Two views of the anatomy and the forces through these structures which entrap
the left palatine bone.
Illustration IV–10

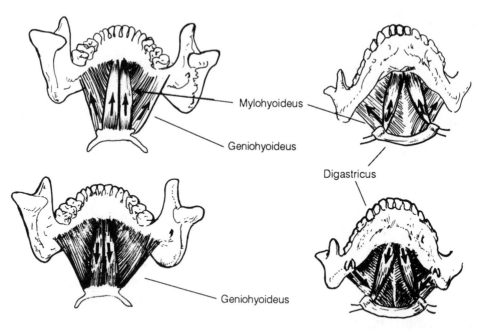

Functional anatomy of the suprahyoid musculature. All of these muscles serve to retract the mandible when the hyoid bone is fixed by the infrahyoid and pharyngeal constrictor muscles. Hypertonus of these suprahyoid muscles then serve to impact the mandibular condyle into the posterior aspect of the temporomandibular joint fossa. This situation may unfavorably affect the retrodiscal elastic tissues.
Illustration IV–11

Once I realized what had happened, I put my finger under the zygoma inside the mouth and grasped the external part of the zygoma with my thumb. I then used several ounces of force to move the zygoma laterally. This allows more maxillary movement and some increased palatine movement. The symptoms abated as long as I held the zygoma. When I got the palatine partially released all the symptoms abated temporarily. Relief continued for a few days after I let go. This was progress, but we still had a distance to travel.

Once you have finished the palatines (at least for that session) go back and rebalance the hard palate in flexion and extension with the sphenoid. Also (please) rebalance the mandible with focus on moving it anterior to accommodate the anterior repositioning you have done with the hard palate complex by the decompression of the hard palate in relationship to the sphenoid.[16]

---

[16] See *CranioSacral Therapy*, Chapter XII, for a more basic description of these maxillary, vomer and palatine hard palate techniques.

THE SOFT TISSUES, HYOID AND FACE

Now let's consider the tissues that help you get deeper into the parts of the mouth, face and throat. These are the tissues that open the gates for more effective SomatoEmotional Release, therapeutic imagery and dialogue.

The hyoid bone has long been a focus of fascination for me. It is held in its precarious position by muscles coming from several directions. There, muscles that come from below attach to the sternoclavicular complex. It, in turn, has muscles that run posteriorly and attach to the median raphe at the back of the neck. It also has muscles that run anteriorly and anterolaterally. These muscles contribute to the floor of the mouth. They then attach to the mandible. It also provides attachment for the digastricus and the stylohyoideus muscles that arise from the mastoid and styoid processes of the temporal bones respectively. The digastricus passes through a ligamentous sling attached to the superior aspect of the body of the hyoid bone

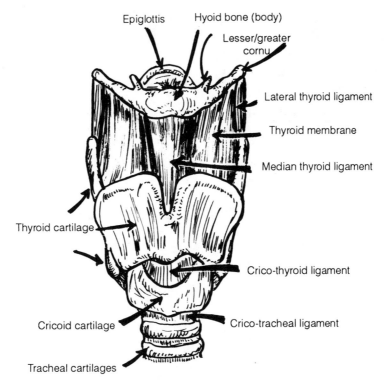

Anterior view of the structures of the throat with the hyoid bone above and the tracheal cartilages below. Structural dysfunction here is frequently secondary to emotionally related suppression of vocal expression— topics about which the patient has been unable to talk, yell or scream.
Illustration IV–12a

and then its anterior belly continues and attaches to the forward part of the mandible. The omohyoid muscle also deserves special note: It connects the inferior aspect of the hyoid body to the clavicle and first rib via a ligamentous sling, then it continues to attach to the upper scapula.[17]

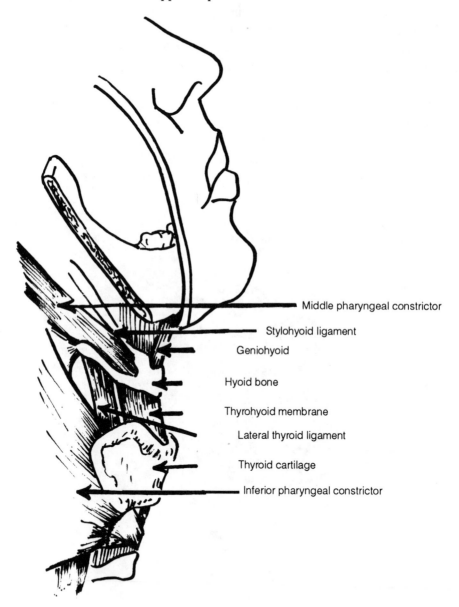

Middle pharyngeal constrictor

Stylohyoid ligament

Geniohyoid

Hyoid bone

Thyrohyoid membrane

Lateral thyroid ligament

Thyroid cartilage

Inferior pharyngeal constrictor

Side view of those throat structures which are considered in the anterior release techniques.
Illustration IV–12b

[17] See *CranioSacral Therapy II, Beyond the Dura*, pp. 130 – 143, for more detailed functional and structural anatomy of the hyoid bone and its related muscles and other structures.

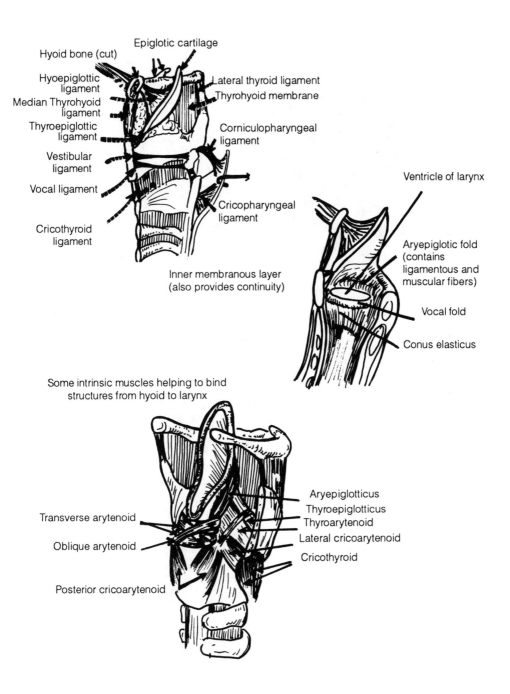

Detailed anatomy of the throat structures.
Illustration IV–12c

Frontal section through the cavity of the larynx

Epiglottic cartilage

Vestibule of larynx

Hyoid bone

Quadrangular membrane

Thyrohyoid membrane

Thyrohyoid

Ryngeal ventricle

Ayrepiglotticus

Vocalis

Thyroid cartilage

Lateral cricoarytenoid

Sternohyoid

Cricothyroid

Inferior pharygeal constrictor

Cricoid cartilage

Cricotracheal ligament

Posterior median (pharyngeal) raphe: is continuous with connective tissue that passes posterior to the spinous processes of the cervical vertebrae

Superior constrictor

Middle constrictor

Hyoid

Inferior constrictor

Posterior views of the throat structures in question—cutaway view above, attachment of the pharyngeal constrictor muscles below.
Illustration IV–12d

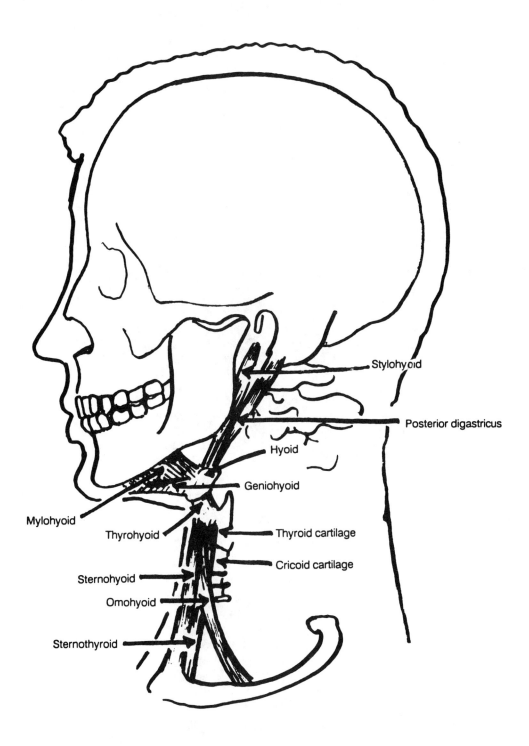

Supra and infrahyoid muscles from the side.
Illustration IV–12e

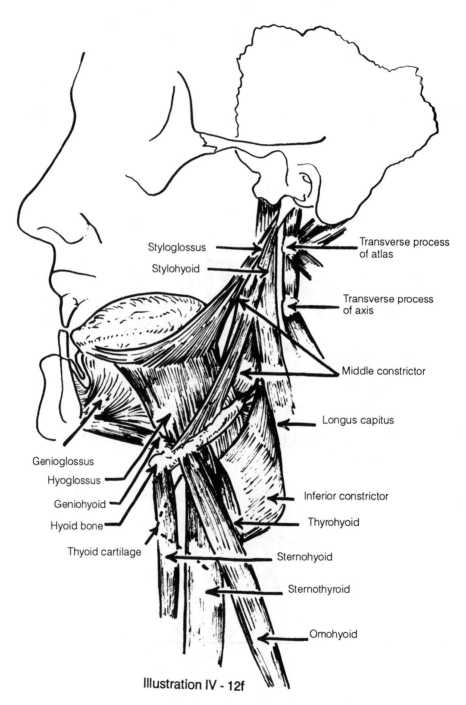

Illustration IV - 12f

Anatomy of the muscles that attach to and influence the hyoid bone.
Illustration IV–12f

All these muscles serve to retract the mandible when the hyoid bone is flexed by the infrahyoid and pharyngeal constrictor muscles. Hypertonus of these suprahyoid muscles then serve to impact the mandibular condyle into the posterior aspect of the temporomandibular joint fossa. This situation may unfavorably affect the retrodiscal elastic tissues.

A quick look at functional geometry of this anatomy reveals that when stabilized, the hyoid offers an anchor to those muscles that can pull the mandible posteriorly in a very powerful way. These muscles are the geniohyoideus, the mylohyoideus and to some extent the digastricus, although the digastricus serves to elevate the hyoid bone as well as retract the mandible. The major stabilization of the hyoid, to anchor it against the anteriorly and slightly superiorly directed force of those muscles (geniohyoideus, mylohyoideus and anterior belly of the digastricus) that form the floor of the mouth, is principally by the constructor pharyngeus medius muscles that attach to the hyoid bone, go around the neck and attach to the median raphe posteriorly. This raphe is related via tough connective tissue to the spinous processes of the cervical vertebrae. Thus when the muscles of the floor of the mouth are contracted, the constrictor pharyngeal muscles must contract to counterbalance and maintain reasonable hyoid bone position. When these posterior stabilizing muscles remain chronically overactive, they produce restriction and dysfunction of the upper cervical vertebrae. When you release the muscles of the floor of the mouth, you can very definitely feel the releasing of the upper cervical vertebrae as the necessity for posterior stabilization of the hyoid bone is reduced.

Also keep in mind that the hyoid bone and the thyroid cartilage just below are closely connected by membrane, ligament and muscle. Wherever the hyoid bone goes, it urges the thyroid cartilage to go along. And since the larynx (voice box) is connected to all the thyrohyoid ligaments, it also feels the stress when the hyoid is pulled in one direction or another or immobilized by muscular hypertonicity. Patients with hyoid problems often find it difficult to talk in a relaxed way. It takes effort and the voice sounds strained.

The next series of techniques are designed to relax and release the muscles that attach to the hyoid bone. In so doing, we also beneficially affect the thyroid cartilage and the larynx. This greatly improves the ability of patients/clients to express themselves verbally and vocally. It also allows for improvement of (fifth) throat chakra function. The order of presentation is not rigid, but in general I have found that when used in the sequence as given below, there seems to be a quicker response.

I like to release the tissues that contribute to the floor of the mouth initially. These tissues include the mylohyoideus muscles, the geniohyoideus muscles and the anterior bellies of the digastricus muscles. The technique requires both hands, one inside the mouth and the other outside the mouth. I use one finger, either index or middle, of the internal hand to reach toward my external finger, again either index or third, during this releasing technique.

Gently place the outside fingertip on the soft tissue just posterior to the angle of the mandible. Now very slowly and gently insert the internal finger beneath the tongue on the medial (internal) side of the mandible on the same side of the patient as you placed your external finger. Slowly and respectfully move your internal finger tip toward your external finger tip. Allow time for the tissues to relax and accommodate your internal finger. (This may be the first time a finger has ever gone into these places.) Blend your finger with the tissues. Do not allow your finger to be a foreign object. As you blend your finger with the patient's tissues, put an intention of relaxation through your finger AND put an intention to touch your external finger through your internal finger. Make a closed energy loop between your internal and your external fingers. You will feel the tissues respond by softening and allowing your internal finger deeper into their reaches. After these tissues have released, slowly and gently follow the internal, inferior border of the mandible with both the internal and external fingers from its angle to its anterior midline at the symphysis menti (point of the chin.) As you move along this mandibular border, continue to blend with the soft tissues that attach to the mandible. Continue to visualize generic healing energy passing from your internal fingertip toward your external finger. Move slowly enough for the patient's tissues to relax and accommodate your finger.

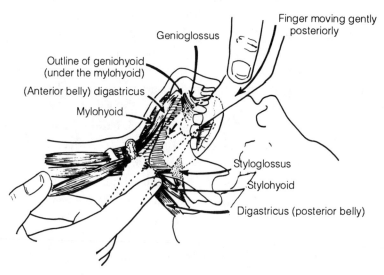

Finger positions used for the release of the suprahyoid musculature and other soft tissues. Note the external fingertip at the left is just posterior to the angle of the mandible while the internal finger at top right is very gently reaching for the external fingertip.
Illustration IV–13

When you encounter resistance or a band of restriction, stay with it. Wait until it releases and disappears. Frequently, you will meet small bands of contracted muscle or fiber that appear to extend from the mandible medially toward the hyoid bone. When you meet one of these, blend with it, broadcast your relaxation into it through your fingers and wait for it to respond before you move on.

Now repeat the procedure on the other side. Change your internal hand to external and vice versa. Make your entry. Blend. Broadcast your kind and helping intention. Connect your two fingers with generic, healing energy. Move slowly and gently from the region posterior to the mandibular angle to the point of the chin.

After you have done this technique once on both sides, do it again on both sides. The first time you do it, there will usually be much obvious discomfort. The second time it will be much more comfortable and the tissues will feel much better to you and about you. I suggest that the second time through the process you make yourself aware that as you are working posterior to the angle of the mandible, you are influencing the stylohyoideus and the posterior belly of the digastricus muscles. Relaxation of these muscles will free the temporal bones to move more easily into external rotation. The stylohyoideus attaches to the styloid process of the temporal bone and the posterior belly of the digastricus attaches on the internal aspect of the mastoid process of the temporal bone. Your awareness of this anatomy and your intention to help these structures relax will hasten the actual happening.

As you move your fingers a little anterior from the angle of the mandible, you are working through the mylohyoid muscle that contributes the majority of the muscle to the floor of the mouth. Be aware that between your fingers is a muscle that directly connects the mandible to the hyoid bone and, via this connection, exercises great influence upon the throat and the voice box. Therefore, it has a great deal to do with one's ability to be vocally expressive. About halfway from the mandibular angle to the point of the mandibular chin you will feel a salivary gland duct. Don't wait there forever, in hope that this duct will totally disappear. It will soften and feel relaxed, but it will still be there unless you have more energy than I have.

As you approach the anterior extreme of the floor of the mouth, the tissues thicken. Be aware that you are encountering the geniohyoideus and the anterior belly of the digastricus muscles. Get them nice and soft and relaxed, but don't expect them to disappear so that the thickness of the floor of the mouth anteriorly is the same as it is more laterally and posteriorly.

The next technique to do is to re-enter the posterior reaches of the lower part of the mouth under the tongue. This time I will use only an internal finger. After inserting as far back as I can, using very gentle persuasion, I position my finger so that the palmar side is facing the root of the tongue. Then I very gently direct a small force and a large intention into the root of the tongue. In this technique, you will be approaching the hyoglossus muscles that attach to the hyoid bone and extend superiorly to contribute to the tongue. When the hyoglossus muscles contract, they bring the tongue back toward the floor of the mouth. As you move forward you will influence the genioglossus muscle of the tongue that exercises further control on the tongue movement in terms of protrusion and retraction. Release these muscles from both sides twice, just as you did in the floor of the mouth. I want to thank Benjamin Shield for my introduction to these techniques during a Rolfing session in which he was the Rolfer and I was the Rolfee. The description shows significant modification of the techniques, but he planted the seeds. Thank you, Benjamin.

While you are in the mouth, you may as well treat the gums. These poor gums are continually battered and beaten when chewing. They have been injected with Novocain by dentists. They have been probed and abraded by dental hygienists and so on. Give them a chance to release. Most gums are full of Energy Cysts simply because the patient is usually full of fear and anxious anticipation when any work is done in the mouth. To release the gums, I just place an external hand on the side of the face with my palm either over the maxillary gum region or the

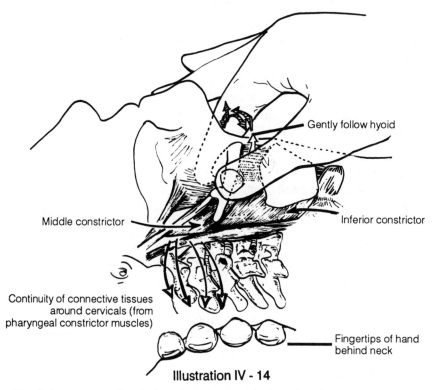

Gently follow hyoid

Middle constrictor

Inferior constrictor

Continuity of connective tissues
around cervicals (from
pharyngeal constrictor muscles)

Fingertips of hand
behind neck

Illustration IV - 14

Hand placement and technique for release of the hyoid and its attached pharyngeal
constrictor muscles. See text.
Illustration IV–14

mandibular gum region depending on whether I'll be working on the upper or lower gum. With an internal finger, I begin on the internal aspect of the gum posteriorly and slowly move forward to the incisor region of the gum. You have the gum between your internal finger and your external hand. Go slowly. Broadcast energy from your external hand to your internal finger or vice versa if the body tells you that it would prefer it that way. As you encounter Energy Cysts or restricted areas, stay there until they release. Do this technique on both sides, upper and lower gums twice just as you did the floor of the mouth and the tongue.

I don't usually evaluate the teeth now, but it can be done at this point. Intuitively it seems better to me to complete the hyoid and throat releases first, then return to the teeth. I think this is because the teeth are a little more subtle in their messages to the therapeutic facilitator. It is probably better to clear background noise from the hyoid and throat so that these subtle tooth messages are not obscured by noise.

To release the pharyngeal constrictor muscles, which retract the hyoid posteriorly, I very gently place a finger and a thumb of one hand on the lateral aspects of the hyoid bone and hold it. Then I place my other hand under the supine patient's

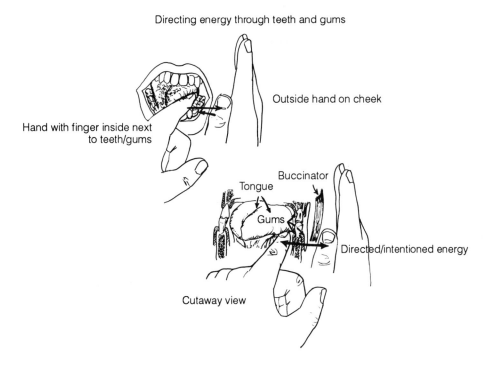

Finger and hand positions used for the release of Energy Cysts from the gums and teeth.
Illustration IV–15

neck so that I am holding the upper cervical vertebrae with my index finger, my middle finger and the side of my palm and my thumb. Now, I strongly intention release and follow wherever it goes during its self-correction process. You will experience a great release when the technique is complete.

For the infrahyoid muscles (omohyoid, sternohyoid and thyrohyoid), place one hand gently over the throat and the other under the middle cervicals. Strongly intention release. Follow the self-corrective process. Encourage it whenever it needs a little boost and wait for the release to occur. (This is almost too easy isn't it? Enjoy. I'm sure that Nature intended it to be that way.)

Once I accomplish these releases, I move back into the mouth to evaluate and release Energy Cysts, emotion and trauma from the teeth. To evaluate the teeth, I

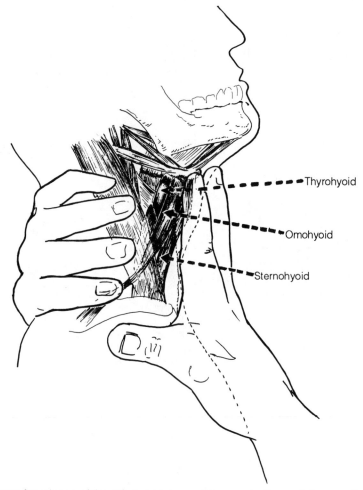

Hand placement for release of the infrahyoid musculature and other soft tissues. See text.
Illustration IV–16

have patients open their mouths comfortably. I then place the palmar surface of two of my fingers on the biting surfaces of either the upper or lower molars and premolars on both sides. You will do both upper and lower ultimately. I don't believe it matters much which ones you do first.

As you rest your fingers on these biting surfaces you may gradually become aware that a certain tooth or teeth have more or less energy than the others. When this becomes clear, I place a fingertip on both the medial and lateral sides of the tooth in question. Then I intention a release and wait for it to happen. After a minute or so, the tooth will autonomously begin to reposition itself in the maxilla or the mandible, depending on where you are working. Follow this activity to the release which represents the end of the treatment for that tooth. Then re-evaluate and work with the next tooth that gets your attention.

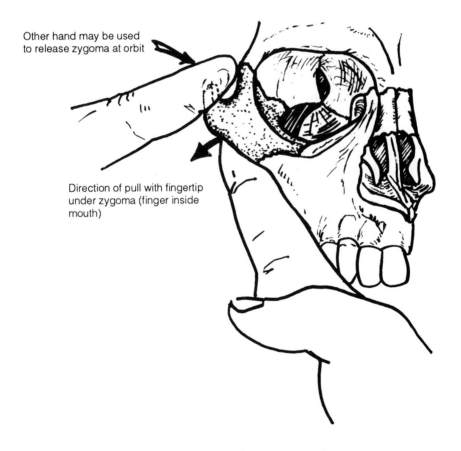

Other hand may be used to release zygoma at orbit

Direction of pull with fingertip under zygoma (finger inside mouth)

Hand position used for release of zygoma. See text.
Illustration IV–17

To evaluate the canine and incisor teeth, I hold two or three at a time between my thumb and index or middle fingers. The tooth or teeth that need attention will jump out at you and begin their therapeutic repositioning. When this happens, focus on the tooth in question. Energize it and follow it to its end release. When no more teeth show that they want to reposition and release, you are finished with the teeth. I re-evaluate two or three times before I assume completion of the treatment of the teeth. Take your time, it may take a minute or two for the message from a tooth to break through into your conscious awareness.

(If you have a colleague with you, it is fun to have one of you observe arcing patterns on the total body as the other does the tooth work. This exercise will offer you a lot of valuable opportunity to gain insight into the relationship between the teeth and the rest of the body.)

There is another evaluative process I like to do before leaving the mouth, face and throat. This technique probes the function of the zygoma, its sutural relationships to the temporal, the maxilla and the frontal and its contribution to the orbit. In this technique I gently and with sensitivity to tissue response, place a finger between the maxilla (on its outer aspect) and the zygoma. Feel the zygoma move. I would like it to go up and out. If it doesn't, I'll put a little pressure on it over a period of time. This will usually be enough to re-establish its mobility. If the resistance is greater than can be effectively treated by this finger, then I grasp the orbital rim of the zygoma with my thumb. I now hold the bone between my finger (in the mouth) and my thumb (on the rim of the orbit). Gently traction the zygoma in an anterolateral direction. This will decompress the sutures and the orbit of the eye. I repeat, use a small force for a longer time; a longer duration with a much smaller force is much preferable to a stronger force over a shorter duration because you will not recruit tissue resistance and/or defenses, nor will you induce secondary dysfunction.

In 1990, I had the privilege of working with a 26-year-old female patient who had suffered a rear end collision some four years earlier. She did not feel that she was severely injured and declined medical attention at the time of the accident. Now, four years and many doctors later, she arrived at our Institute with extreme, unrelenting throat pain and anterior cervical muscle spasm. She had a diagnosis of atypical torticollis in her portfolio of medical opinions and laboratory reports. I don't understand the mechanics of her situation completely, but what I saw was the most clear-cut case of suprahyoid and pharyngeal muscle contracture ever. There seemed to be no emotional component. After four sessions, involving the use of the techniques that release the floor of the mouth and the pharyngeal constrictor muscles as described above, she is completely pain free and rehabilitated. It is one of the purest cases I have ever seen.

Keep in mind, however, that there are really very few cases this pure. The great majority of patients, once the mouth and throat have been opened will begin to express themselves and their feelings much more readily. In fact, they may begin to express either while you are still releasing or right after. Once it starts, let it go, don't try to inhibit the flow of energy that comes out of the mouth and throat. It may involve words or it may involve just sounds and screams.

After this initial expressive release is complete, I like to do throat chakra work and to re-evaluate and integrate the Vector/Axis system (as described in Chapter III). To accomplish the chakra, you simply place one hand under the neck and the other gently over the throat. Tune in and feel the energy. Sense the chakra. It may be blocked, turning counterclockwise instead of clockwise and so on. Offer it the chance to normalize and give it that intention. Chances are, it will. Then feel what a normally functioning throat chakra feels like. It will turn clockwise and will lift your hand off the throat. There may be one in the midline or there may be two smaller chakras, one on each side of the Adam's apple. Both situations are quite functional.[18]

Chances are, the next time you see the patient, he or she will tell you how they have told people things they had been wanting to tell them for a long time. Or they found themselves singing in the shower. Or they can now cry or laugh and so on and so on and so on.

It is really very good work. Take your time, be meticulous and enjoy observing the results.

---

[18]   See *CranioSacral Therapy II, Beyond the Dura*, pp. 229 – 230, for a description of chakras and how to treat them.

Chapter V
Therapeutic Image
and Dialogue

IMAGINATION, FANTASY AND TALKING TO YOURSELF

It is bedtime. The light in my room is off but my bedroom door is ajar and some light from the hallway is coming in. Mom has tucked me in and kissed me goodnight. She doesn't understand about the monster in my closet. The monster always tries to get me when the light in my room is turned off and I'm supposed to sleep. He is looking out of the closet now and I can see his yellow eyes shining. He wants to kidnap me and take me away forever. He starts to come out of the closet. I'm so scared. My heart is pounding out of my chest and I can't make a sound. And just in the nick of time, my angel Jennifer appears on the windowsill, all shiny and sparkly. All she has to do is point her magic wand at the monster and he stops in his tracks. Then he starts slowly to back into the closet where he stays. He looks at Jennifer and makes ugly faces at her.

Jennifer says, "John, don't be so afraid, I'll always be here to protect you." I still can't make a sound or move a muscle but my heart quiets down a little. Jennifer comes closer and spreads some magic dust on me so I can talk and move. Jennifer says again, "John, I really will protect you from the monster."

And I say, "But what if you don't get here in time and the monster takes me into the closet with him? He has a secret tunnel from the closet to Monsterland and if he gets me there I'll never get back."

Jennifer replies "John, please believe me. I really won't ever let the monster take you away or hurt you even a little bit."

"But Jennifer, what if he sneaks out of the closet when you aren't watching and takes me where you never could find me?"

"John," it's my mother's voice as she enters my bedroom, "are you talking about monsters again? And who are you talking to?" Mom turns on my bedroom light. "See there isn't anyone here. Who are you talking to?"

I try to tell Mom about the monster in the closet who comes out to get me when the bedroom light is off. Mom says, "But you're still here. The monster didn't get you. And look! There isn't any monster in the closet," as she opens the closet door and turns on the light. I can't look, I'm afraid to look in my closet.

"And who were you talking to about the monsters?" Mom says.

"I was talking to my angel, Jennifer. She saved me. She scared the monster away."

"That's enough foolishness, go to sleep, it's late. Forget about monsters and angels. There isn't anyone here. You are letting your imagination run away with you. You've got to stop imagining things."

I feel humiliated and frustrated. Mom never believes me about the monsters or about Jennifer. Why won't she believe me?

For my fifth birthday, a dream came true. I got a 12-bass accordion and beginner's lessons at the Wurlitzer Music Studio in Detroit. When I was three we

New Year's Eve party at our house and a man came over with his accordion—a "stomach squeezer," I called it. I was entranced. Dad bought me a little toy concertina to placate me until I was old enough to get a real accordion and lessons at Wurlitzer. I was so excited. After a few lessons, I started to learn some basic, familiar songs like "Jingle Bells" and "La Golendrina." In a very short time I was adding a few little creative licks of my own to these songs.

Each time I demonstrated my own creative improvisation my teacher rapped the music stand with her baton. She told me to play the music just as it was written. Soon, I began to stand up for myself, telling her it sounded better my way. She would then tell me that it would take some years before I could write my own music. Until then, I had to play it like it was written. The accordion lost a lot of its appeal when I had to do it strictly her way.

Fortunately, Dad saw the problem and wisely intervened. He gave me a dollar with which I could buy three sheets of popular music if I got a gold star for my lesson each week. Once I had the sheet music with the words and the melody, I could sing and play the song any way I wanted to. Not many aspiring musicians have the kind of father who will nurture individual creativity in contradiction to the system. I was extremely fortunate.

I was in third grade. It was spring. Spring fever was upon me. My seat in the classroom was toward the back of the room (because my name starts with "U," pretty far down the alphabet) near the window. All I could think about was outside—how blue the sky was, how billowy and fluffy the clouds were, how warm the sun was. Why did I have to sit here in this classroom able only to dream of outdoors and freedom? Soon my attention was captured by a hawk making circles in the sky as hawks do. I kept watching the hawk as he glided gracefully through the sky. Suddenly I was in an open-cockpit biplane. I followed the hawk doing his circles.

In only a second or two I had become an aviator. I was flying my own airplane. As I followed the hawk, I got closer and closer. Finally I was flying beside him. I asked him what he was doing. He replied that he was practicing to be the world's best flying hawk. I was truly impressed. I asked if he minded if I fly along with him.

He said, "Not at all," and suggested that so long as we were going to fly together I should call him by his first name, Henry. I then told him that my name was John. He said, "Hello John, I'm pleased to meet you."

My grandfather always said, "Likewise I'm sure," so I said, "Henry, it's likewise I'm sure." Suddenly we were good friends.

I told Henry that if he was practicing to be the world's best flying hawk and if I did what he did follow-the-leader style, I could probably became the world's best aviator. Henry thought that made sense and agreed to lead me through the stunts he knew. Soon we were doing loop-the-loops, stalls, dives and figure eights, and I was right on his tail feathers.

As I became more involved in the follow-the-leader exercise, I must have put my arms out like airplane wings and made the appropriate biplane engine roaring noises, because just when I was getting really hot I was brought down to earth by a firm grip and pull on my right ear by my teacher. (In retrospect, she either corrected an external rotation restriction or produced an internal rotation restriction of my right temporal bone.)

"Come back down to earth, young man. That's enough daydreaming. We have work to do. If you don't get finished, you will have to go to summer school," she told me in a stern, no-nonsense voice. I learned right then that fantasy is not allowed in the third grade.

These experiences are similar to those that occur in all our lives. They serve to demonstrate that fantasy, imagination, talking to yourself and so on are all seriously discouraged from very early on, at home and in most school systems. Because success in school depends largely on "paying attention," "being real," memorization and parroting, most parents try to get their children to let go of any embarrassing fantasy life at a fairly early age. Fantasy just isn't productive. There may even be something "wrong" with the child who overindulges in fantasy.

I had occasion to work with and develop a rather deep friendship with a world renowned psychic who stayed in the closet about her talents until she was about 40 years old. Why? Because during the flu epidemic of 1918 when she was a very little girl, she went around the neighborhood wearing a little nurse's hat, and she put her hands on flu victims' foreheads. Those people that she touched got better. They told her mother about it. Her mother spanked her and told her not to do that any more. It was bad. It wasn't normal to be able to do that. Only witches did those kinds of things.

As therapeutic facilitators who make use of therapeutic imagery and dialogue in our work, it is this kind of negative indoctrination that we have to overcome in many of our patients/clients. After all, what is therapeutic imagery but active imagination, and dialogue is talking to yourself. Usually, if you talk to yourself enough you get to spend some time in a rubber room and (perhaps) get some drugs to inhibit your creative images and to stop you from talking to them if they do form. Now here you are as a therapeutic facilitator trying to convince the patient/client's brow-beaten, insulted and inhibited creative, imaginative energies that it is safe to come out and show themselves and let us see what they can do.

That these talents are present in most of us is demonstrated by the wonderful success of Bill Cosby, Whoopi Goldberg, Robin Williams, Billy Crystal and several other entertainers who make it okay to visualize a chicken heart that is eating Chicago or a kid named Fat Albert flattening a whole Buck Buck team or a Valley Girl or a sperm or a silly old man on a park bench. Audiences love to use their imaginations in settings where it is permissible. It becomes your job as therapeutic facilitator to convince the patient/client that it is also okay to have an image of a very wise old physician who lives inside them. A physician who can present in any form that they choose. This Inner Physician may show himself or herself as a dove or a lump of coal, as an angel or as anything else. The Inner Physician may not present itself visually. It may present as a voice, as a smell or as a feeling. However a patient's Inner Physician chooses to present itself, the patient/client must be helped to understand that this wise being can provide good advice, knows and understands the problems and can be of inestimable help in finding solutions. The patient must also be brought to understand that if done carefully and politely, a dialogue can be established between their Inner Physician, their conscious awareness and yourself as the therapeutic facilitator. Once you speak directly to the patient's Inner Physician, the option is available to keep your conversation with that Inner Physician confidential and not immediately available to the patient's conscious awareness. I do this only at the request of the Inner Physician, however, or if it occurs spontaneously.

Even more ridiculous, a symptom such as a back pain may be asked to present itself. Upon my request, my own chronic back pain presented itself as a boomerang. It spoke with me and told me about itself and its purpose. It told me that it only hurt me when it was inflated. It told me that what inflated it was anger. It led me to understand that anger will always come back at me like a boomerang and give me a back pain. I understood. Now when I have that back pain, I search inside to see what I'm angry about. When I find it and discharge it, the pain leaves. It is amazing how often you are subliminally angry. I thank my boomerang for letting me know.

This productive use of imagination, creativity, imagery and internal dialogue flies in the face of what has been taught and conditioned into so many of us. We are conditioned to "get real" and "stay real." Therefore, the most difficult part of therapeutic imagery and dialogue may be initiating it and making it credible. The therapeutic facilitator has to be a good salesperson in this instance. To sell, you must believe in your product. If you are embarrassed, inhibited or skeptical of the efficacy of therapeutic imagery and dialogue, have someone work with you until you are comfortable with its concepts and uses. You may also discover that the patient requires constant and literal reassurance and support for the significance and credibility of what he or she is doing. This reassurance can be through your words, with your tone of voice, with your touch and with your intention. These modes may be used concurrently, interchangeably and individually as it seems appropriate at any given moment in any given session.

WHAT'S QUANTUM PHYSICS GOT TO DO WITH IT?

Quantum physics is the outgrowth of the seed planted by Max Planck in 1900. Planck proposed the Quantum Theory at about that time. His proposition puts forth the concept that there is no such thing as a pure continuum in the physical world. Energy, motion, mass all exist in tiny parcels or quanta. These quanta are so small that they give the appearance of continuity, but when viewed in minute detail, all things are made up of tiny pieces, even motion. For example, an oscillator cannot gain or lose energy along a continuum. It gains or loses its energy in discrete amounts, which Planck termed "quanta." Each quantum is considered to have its own specific amount of energy. In electromagnetic radiation, the quantum is the photon.

In 1905 Einstein used Planck's Quantum Theory to explain the photoelectric effect. In 1913 Bohr used Planck's theory to explain the atomic spectra. In 1933 Erwin Schrödinger was awarded the Nobel Prize for the development of the wave equation which gave birth to quantum mechanics as it is today. Quantum mechanics is the science that describes electron and small particle behavior. Quantum electrodynamics is a further extension that deals with the behavior of charged particles in a quantized field. It is used to explain interactions between electrons, positrons and radiation. All the quantum sciences are the progeny of Max Planck's insight that led him to the formulation of the Quantum Theory. What's Quantum Theory and quantum physics got to do with imagery and dialogue? We'll see.

From 1960 through 1964, I had the distinct privilege of working as a Teaching and Research Fellow for a very brilliant man named Stacy F. Howell. He was a biochemist, and I was his first and only Fellow. He was near retirement, so he used me as a sounding board for many thoughts and ideas he had developed during his lifetime. Dr. Howell had a huge stack of handwritten notes on the subject of size. He proposed as food for thought that a molecule may be a mini-model of a galaxy and that an atomic nucleus might be a mini-model of a sun with the electrons analogous to the planets circling that sun. He further proposed that these analogous relationships existed between all things; the only variable was size. He proposed that each particle was a hologram of the whole of which that particle was a fragment. He lectured to me and at me for hours on this subject. The cell was a mini-human being and the electron was a mini-earth circling its nucleus as earth circles the sun.

Letting our imaginations stretch a little, we can consider electrons and their possible analogous relationship to people, minds, imaginations and images. When electrons are shot from electron guns, as in your television set, they seem able to behave as either particles or waves. Whether the electron behaves as a particle or a wave seems to depend on the means with which we choose to observe it. When we fire electrons through a slit into a cloud chamber they seem to behave as particles.

That is, they travel through the mist inside the chamber and leave a trail visible to the human observer. On the other hand, if we shoot electrons through the same slit at a photographic film, the results suggest that waves are striking the film—from whence the argument about whether electrons are particles or waves comes.

This apparent discrepancy regarding the nature of the electron raises the question in the minds of some theoretical physicists about whether the electron might be both a particle and a wave, depending upon how we choose to observe it. The next question is whether the electron would behave as either or neither a particle or a wave if there were no observer. Perhaps the electron has a consciousness that understands our puzzlement and our need to understand. The electron may wish to accommodate us. Thus, if we decide to look for a particle, the electron acts like a particle. Or if we are looking for a wave it gives us a wave. Sometimes the electrons may be in playful or contrary moods and behave in a way opposite from that which we expect. This seems to happen fairly often. One experiment's results are opposite from another. Are electrons mini-people? Some show you what you want to see and others being contrary, show you just the opposite of what you expect. If electrons are performing for the experimenter in the way that the experimenter expects them to perform, what are the electrons doing when no experiment is in progress? Is there an electron behavioral phenomenon when no one is watching? Or does our watching trigger the behavior?

When your hands perceive something, was it there when your hands weren't there to perceive? I have had many therapists/facilitators tell me about new rhythms they perceive and new vectors that they see. It is both astonishing and sobering. Would these rhythms and vectors be there without the therapeutic facilitator? This sounds like imagination and it sounds like I may be beginning to make a case against the credibility of what we—as hands-on therapists—perceive. Not so. The next and more amazing thing that occurs is that these imagined rhythms and vectors are often used successfully to obtain a positive therapeutic effect.

As I discussed these questions in the spring of 1989, one of the class participants described her experience. She had some difficulty in using and seeing the Vector/Axis system as I had presented it. Being an impulsive, uninhibited, creative type she invented her own vectors and axes. She invented a vector to serve whatever purpose she felt she needed. Lo and behold her imagined/invented/improvised vectors worked for her and her patient/client. A positive therapeutic result was obtained. She states that she has repeated this process many times with a very high percentage of success. I believe her.

When we work with a patient/client, we may get what we expect or we may get just the opposite. Just as there may be some contrary electrons, we may have some contrary people who give us contrary responses. If we expect to feel the craniosacral system, we'll feel it. If we expect the manipulation of this craniosacral system to yield positive therapeutic effect, it will—except in the case of contrary response.

If we can get an image with the patient of what we truly and mutually want, we can have our wish. Perhaps, as with electrons and with people, reality occurs when we perceive it. If this is true when we image something, we make it happen. Used correctly, therapeutic imaging with dialogue is an extremely effective therapeutic modality.

That's what quantum physics has to do with it.

THE THERAPEUTIC IMAGE

The therapeutic image may present itself either spontaneously (if there is such a thing) or upon your request. In either case, when a significant image presents itself to the patient, the Significance Detector—the sudden stoppage of the craniosacral rhythm—will tell you so.

As you recall, the Significance Detector is the sudden stoppage of the craniosacral rhythm. When you are just working with no conversation and not following a body position (as you would in SomatoEmotional Release) and the craniosacral rhythm suddenly stops, this is the Significance Detector. It could stop in extreme flexion or extreme extension or anywhere between. It will often stop with an extreme degree of tension held in the system. This is in contrast to the relaxed state of the craniosacral system when a Still Point occurs.

1. *The Unsolicited Image*

When this sudden stop occurs, it is the Significance Detector's signal that something good is happening inside, that it has either arrived in the patient's conscious awareness or is just outside the boundary and is about to enter. At the instant you feel the "stop," ask the patient/client, "What is in your mind right now?" Tell the individual not to worry about how silly it may seem, just ask him/her to tell you what was there at the instant you asked the question. Usually, the patient/client has some difficulty in answering you. (It is a little like playing musical chairs. The music stops, and you awkwardly scramble for a chair; but with practice, you get better. Soon you know precisely where you are in relation to each chair when the music stops. The same is true of patients/clients.) Initially, he/she may not be able to tell you what was going on at a precise instant, but with practice the patient/client will improve. It may be like a dream, gone from awareness in a fraction of a second.

If a patient/client can't tell you when you ask, be sure that you are very kind about it. Let him or her know that it is common for the instantaneous content to escape. But let him or her know that you may ask again if you get a sense from his/her body—you can explain the Significance Detector if you wish—that the nonconscious may be bringing into awareness something that could be helpful. Remember, the nonconscious mind has heard your comments. It also has tentatively offered the tip of the iceberg. You are telling the nonconscious that you are ready to receive its message and would it please try to communicate to you. I suspect that these verbally unsolicited messages begin to come through because the nonconscious part of the patient senses your touch and the open, helping, sincere attitude that it conveys. The nonconscious part tentatively projects toward you with the hope that you are sympathetic and that the healing process may develop.

After a time or two, when patients are unable to tell you what is in their minds at a specific instant, they will begin to come up with something. Their ability will improve with repetition. What they perceive may not be a visual image. It may be a voice, a feeling or a sense that something is there. I have had several cases where the initial unsolicited image was the smell of ether. Most patients have to be encouraged to tell you about this sensation because they think it is silly and it is not what they are looking for. But if you follow this olfactory perception, for example, it will usually lead into the reprocessing of a previous surgical experience.

Most often it has been the 40-plus-year-old adult going back to reprocess a tonsillectomy. They often have to deal with issues of desertion by parents, impending death by breathing ether through a mask, assault by a doctor or—frequently— being lied to about the pain and, therefore, feeling betrayed. Each case is very individual, but many people initially seem to enter the process by smelling ether. It is not rare for the therapeutic facilitator to smell ether right along with the patient as the experience and its attendant feelings unfold.

When this initial, unsolicited image presents itself and the patient is able to hold onto some part of it, you must do everything in your power to help maintain contact with the part of the nonconscious that is presenting this image to you both. Softly and gently try to get the patient to provide more details about the image. With each detail the communication line is opened further. The rapport between you, the patient's conscious awareness and the nonconscious part that has made the initial communication gesture are strengthened. Ask about size, shape, color, odor, sound, texture, anything you can think of to ask will strengthen conscious/ nonconscious rapport. Ask the patient how he/she feels in the presence of this image. Encourage the process with soft, simple urgings such as "go on" and "tell me more." One of my favorites is, "I'm not sure I understand. Can you help me to understand better what it is that you mean?" This lets patients/clients know you are really trying, helps to dispel the usually troublesome therapist/patient hierarchy and really makes them part of the process i.e., they know something you don't know.

Be there with patients as they further describe their imaging experience. Blend and meld with them through your hands. Image to yourself what they describe. The more you can see of what they see, smell what they smell, hear what they hear, feel what they feel, sense what they sense in every way possible, the more effectively the therapeutic process will progress.

2. Soliciting an Image
There are many ways to solicit an image. The patient/client or the therapeutic/ facilitator can ask that an Inner Physician, an inner advisor, an inner wisdom, a higher self, a pain, a disease, a tumor or anything else to "please" come into conscious awareness and communicate. I like the patient to use the plural pronoun

"us" right from the start because it opens the door for you, the therapeutic facilitator, to be included in the imagery and dialogue process from the beginning. Then later, when you may wish to dialogue directly with the image, you are already at least partially accepted and included in the process. Dialoguing with the image while using the patient's conscious awareness as an intermediary can become awkward and cumbersome.

When you request an image to present itself your patient/client must be clear that it may assume a totally unexpected form. It is best to have no expectation. The patient must be continually reassured that any and every image is important. None are silly. The patient must be encouraged to describe whatever occurs. You have the Significance Detector working for you. When you and your patient/client make a request for an image to communicate or come forward, you simply wait quietly until the craniosacral rhythm abruptly stops. When it does, ask the individual what is there and what is sensed. (You know something is there, you just have to get the patient to tell you about it.)

If the patient begins to describe an image and the craniosacral rhythm has not stopped, you should recognize that this is probably not a significant image. DO NOT, I repeat, DO NOT say that to patients/clients. Encourage them to work with this image for awhile. When you encounter this kind of resistance go with it. Don't set up an adversarial situation. Repeat your request or take a little rest. You might begin again with a new and different request. After a few non-significant trials an image that stops the craniosacral rhythm will usually occur. If not, it may be best to do just bodywork for the rest of that session. Try imagery again the next visit. Be patient, work within the patient's ground rules as much as is possible. Don't impose your wishes and expectations on the patient.

Another possibility is that as you pursue the non-significant image the Significance Detector will suddenly tell you that something important has just come up and you need to follow it. This sometimes feels to me as though the patient's nonconscious is testing my sincerity.

Once you establish the image's presence, begin the dialogue. At first I like to simply chat with the image, get friendly and let the image know me. Help the image feel at ease. For example I might say, "Hi, my name is John. I'm trying to help (the patient by name) get a handle on (the problem). I would really like to talk with you. I have a feeling that you are really smart and could help us understand what is going on. I would like to be your friend, so perhaps you could tell me a name that you would prefer that we call you. (Image tells you its name.) That's a neat name. Have we met before?" Ask about how long the image has been aware of the problem, what it does and so on. Really give the image a chance to express itself. You must be sincerely and genuinely interested. Find out what the image would like, what it might suggest, what it knows about the patient and why the problem is there.

If you are talking with a symptom, find out if it is happy doing what it is doing. The symptom is usually not happy. Find out what would make it happy. Usually the symptom wants to be freed of the responsibility of being the symptom that it is. But it feels an obligation to continue as an active symptom as long as the patient doesn't understand the problem or is unwilling to work toward problem resolution. Now you must get the patient to be aware of the purpose behind the symptom and demonstrate this awareness to the symptom. Next, you must convince both patient and symptom that the patient will begin work toward satisfactory resolution as of right now. Then you have to convince the symptom of the sincerity of the patient and of his or her willingness to work toward satisfactory resolutions.

You may also have to educate the symptom. Frequently, the symptom may not be aware that there is an alternative existence available for it. It thinks it has to make pain and is unable to do anything else. Let it know that if its purpose is accomplished and the patient changes, it can do something that is more fun, something that makes it happy. You may even present this happiness as a reward for good work. Symptoms may not have any idea what "happy" is so you may have to help them understand. Further, the symptom may not understand the impact that it is having on the patient's life. You may need to discuss whether the "punishment fits the crime." Frequently the symptom doesn't realize that the punishment is excessively severe. An example might be—and I have seen this quite often—severe pelvic pain in an adult woman that interferes with normal sexual activity. The pain (symptom) is punishment for fondling her genitalia as an infant or toddler. She may have been told repeatedly that good girls don't do such things. I only have to point out to the symptom that as a child she is only doing something that produces a pleasant sensation. She did not yet have a judgment and moral code about such things. Why are you (the symptom) still punishing her so severely 30 years later? As the therapeutic facilitator you may have to reiterate this rationale a few times but finally the symptom will usually agree that the punishment has been excessively severe and is now inappropriate or at least that the punishment has been sufficient and can stop now. At that juncture, you can probably get the symptom to put its energy into a more constructive project of its own choosing which you will, of course, help it to choose.

In summary:

- An unsolicited image will make itself known through the Significance Detector.
- You or the patient/client may request any image to come into the conscious awareness. When a significant image presents itself the Significance Detector will let you know.

- Images that do not stop the craniosacral rhythm may present. These images should be treated with respect and deference. They frequently lead to more significant material. I look at them as sincerity tests of the therapeutic facilitator by the patient/client's nonconscious.
- Once an image is present, strengthen the communication by asking for details about the image.
- Develop a three-way dialogue—between the image, the patient's conscious awareness and you—whenever possible.
- Develop a relaxed friendly atmosphere with the image.
- Find out the image's name preference.
- Phrase your questions in such a way to encourage positive awareness.
- Find out whatever the image can tell you about its purpose.
- Define the problem.
- Define the roles of the various participants. There may be several ages involved after you get started.
- See what would provide the most happiness for each participant.
- Negotiate compromises and educate all participants toward the most positive outcome for all.
- Once you have reached mutual agreement, obtain promises from all participants. Define the roles of each and set up regular daily meetings between all images and the patient/client's awareness. Problems that arise can be resolved at these meetings.
- It may be helpful to ask the patient/client's conscious awareness to become the symptom and negotiate from this position.

TUMORS

Tumors present a special case for SomatoEmotional Release, Therapeutic Imagery and Dialogue because they can be deadly and frequently they invoke great fear. I have had conversations with many tumors, although there were a few I just couldn't get into a decent conversation. In general, the significant tumor will talk to you if you are gentle, respectful and persuasive. The insignificant tumor is frequently incommunicative and will not talk to you, but the Inner Physician may tell you that this tumor is not significant and, therefore, does not have much to say.

Significant tumors can be either malignant or benign but want to be heard in either case. Solicit their dialogue. Malignant tumors may be aware that they are deadly and see no way out or they may not be aware, or at least they may pretend not to be aware, that continuation of their present activity may be deadly to the host. If the host dies, so does the tumor. Make this fact perfectly clear to the tumor. Sometimes the tumor thinks it will go on living even if the host dies. In many of these cases you will have to introduce the tumor to the real world. You may be able to introduce alternatives to death even if the tumor feels that all is hopeless.

I worked with a tumor a few years ago that had to be convinced it would die when the host died. The tumor, which was a breast cancer, was convinced that it had tried to get the patient to change her lifestyle and that it had failed in this task; therefore, (the tumor reasoned) the woman would be better off dead than alive. The tumor informed me that when its host died it would just move on to someone else who needed "guidance." I had to convince the tumor that if the patient died, the tumor would cease to exist. It would not just go into someone else's body to repeat its cycle.

I also had to convince the tumor that the host did not know what the tumor was trying to tell her; she did not know she was supposed to change her lifestyle, nor did she know in what way her lifestyle should be changed. The "crime" was a rejection of femininity. I took the stance that death was a severe punishment for such a crime. I had to explain fun and happiness to this tumor and convince it that if it would lighten up and allow the patient some time to change, it could perhaps find a happier existence.

I asked the tumor to regress immediately because of the threat to life it posed. The tumor agreed to regress (shrink, involute) for awhile while it watched to see if the host would really change lifestyles. The host did and the tumor is no longer diagnosable by traditional medical methods.

When I dialogue with the tumor, it says it is still there as a seed and can recur anytime this patient deviates from the new and acceptable lifestyle. Now, the patient and her tumor dialogue every morning, so if deviations from what the tumor considers "acceptable" occur, I'm sure there will be negotiation between the tumor and host before dangerous regrowth occurs.

This same patient has cystic mastitis of both breasts. Her Inner Physician says that these multiple benign tumor growths are not of any real significance. She can image them away if she wants to. It makes no difference to her Inner Physician. She is working on the normalization of her cystic fibrotic breast tissue for her comfort and self-esteem, not because this tissue has any deep meaning in her life.

Another recent example of insignificant tumors was in a 67-year-old man who had been doing some very successful therapeutic imagery with his heart. During a routine physical exam he was found to have multiple colon polyps and surgery was scheduled. During one of his visits with me he asked if we could do anything about the polyps. I suggested that we could always explore the possibilities.

We connected with his Inner Physician who told us that the polyps lacked a particular purpose, they just happened because he repeatedly ate and drank substances in the past that acted as bowel irritants. He did not do these things any more, but the lining of his bowel had become chronically irritated over the years. Mucus production had inordinately increased and the bowel lining separated from the underlying muscular wall in several places; polyps formed at these sites of separation. I asked if we could do anything to avoid the necessity for surgical removal and if this would be acceptable. The Inner Physician said for us to go ahead and heal the polyps by focusing a healing light and energy in the bowel.

I placed my hands anterior and posterior on the supine patient's body with the sigmoid colon between them. We mutually conjured up a generic healing light/energy. The energy accumulated and enlarged in magnitude. The light kept changing color. We both saw this simultaneously. Then, the energy dissipated suddenly and the light softened. We knew the work was accomplished.

The patient went for surgery about three weeks later. The surgeon put in the sigmoidoscope and to his bewilderment there were no colon polyps to be found. This case represents an example of benign tumors with no particular significance in his present life. They were simply remnants of his previous lifestyle. I would not attempt this process without permission of the patient's Inner Physician!

EMOTIONS

It has been fairly common in my experience to have a patient who is literally full to the brim with potentially destructive emotion such as anger, hate, guilt, fear, resentment, jealousy or any combination thereof. You can usually feel these emotions as soon as you touch one of these patients/clients. Sometimes you may be hit in the face with it when you enter the treatment room. Some of you may even feel it before you enter the room. Destructive quantities of these emotions have such a way of getting your attention.

I used to think that it was best to discharge these destructive emotions immediately and then look for causes. The next phase would be to focus on turning off the production or generator of the anger or the guilt or other destructive emotion by resolution of the problem.

More recently, it dawned upon me that the energy which comprises these destructive emotions is the same energy that makes up such constructive emotions as love, joy and hope. It, therefore, seems logical that for reasons of conservation of energy within a patient/client and for the enhancement of self-esteem, it is preferable to convert destructive emotion into constructive emotion. Now I usually ask the patient/client's Inner Physician or Inner Wisdom or whomever it is that I am in contact with whether it would be possible and preferable to convert the destructive emotion to constructive emotions, thus conserving its inherent energy. When the answer is "Yes"—and it seems that it is the same about 50 – 60 percent of the time—I proceed along this line, getting as much advice and direction as I can from the patient's Inner Physician.

Slightly less than half the time, the answer is, "No, let's just get it out of here," or words to that effect. In this situation, I most often use my hands to help in the release or extraction process. Usually, I have the patient/client localize the destructive emotion under my hands. Together, we imagine that my hands are magnets that can draw the destructive emotion out of the individual's body. I used to have patients push hard from the inside, but I have come to realize that less physical effort on their part often facilitates the therapeutic process. Now I try to establish a "letting it go" rather than a "pushing it out" attitude.

There are two further issues that I should like to clarify before getting into the actual release and extraction process. First, I like to explain to patients/clients that as soon as the destructive emotion passes out of their bodies we will neutralize it and have it converted to generic energy that can be used for constructive purposes by whoever might need it. This precautionary step serves to allay any concerns about polluting the atmosphere with destructive energy if they let it out of their body. (I have found that many people fall back on martyrdom and convince themselves that it is better for them to keep the bad stuff rather than release it into the atmosphere where it can damage other unsuspecting and innocent victims. You can defuse this line of defense by neutralizing the destructive energy as it leaves the body.)

Second, I like to explain to patients/clients that they do not have to physically act upon the destructive energy as they feel it localize and release. For example, if we are discharging anger, simply let the patient know that he or she will feel angry as the energy precipitates, localizes and concentrates in the selected area of the body in preparation for release. I let patients/clients know that this anger can go directly out through their skin into the atmosphere. It does not have to be acted upon by kicking, screaming, beating on you or trashing your treatment room. They can just let it go and as it releases, they will feel the emotion diminish and disappear.

At this point, I probably should explain my use of the words "destructive" and "constructive" as descriptors for the various emotions that we all feel. I used to describe emotions as "negative" and "positive." Anger, hatred, jealousy, fear, resentment were negative. Joy, love, hope, serenity and the like were positive. I have encountered some confusion using "negative" and "positive" as emotion descriptors.

The negatives were undesirable and the positives were desirable emotions in my view. However, in the next sentence, we might discuss a negatively charged electrical atmosphere that is desirable for good health and function or an accumulation of positive ions in an airplane cabin which becomes detrimental (undesirable) to health and function. So, to avoid confusion, I am using "destructive" and "constructive" as my descriptors for emotions.

I anticipate that some of you are feeling the hair stand up on the back of the neck. You might be saying, "Wait a minute; anger isn't necessarily destructive. It may save your life in an emergency or help you survive later when you need energy to keep going." This is true. Anger might give you the superhuman strength to cripple Hulk Hogan were he to attack you. But when this anger continues, it becomes destructive. Anger is a spender. It demands of your heart, your lungs, your liver, your stomach, your colon, your entire physiology. It allows no quarter for the replacement of what it takes from you. It works just like the sympathetic nervous system. It will save your life in an emergency and keep you going under stress, but it also will hasten your demise. It is destructive when the emergency is over and your life has been spared. Hate, anger, jealousy, fear and guilt will consume and destroy their owner if they maintain an ongoing residence.

I have also heard the argument that guilt and fear contribute to the construct of conscience and, therefore, are "good emotions." True, guilt and fear (of punishment) may prevent you from robbing a bank, stealing a car, embezzling from your boss or killing your spouse's lover. Still, it would be much more healthful—both physically and emotionally—if you did not commit wrongful acts because you love and respect humanity, because you are understanding rather than vengeful, because you tolerate a reasonable amount of unpleasantness that may have befallen you at the hands of others. None of us is perfect. We all need to understand this as we strive to improve. Please tolerate my tendency to sermonize. Anyhow, it seems more appropriate at this time to describe emotions as destructive and constructive rather than negative or positive. I doubt I have to justify to these readers the idea that happiness, joy, hope, serenity and the like are constructive to the whole being.

Clinical observation and experience has demonstrated to my satisfaction that specific emotions accumulate in specific body organs. In large part specific organ-emotion correspondences agree with concepts put forth in traditional Chinese literature and in acupuncture. My first exposure to the idea that specific organs collect and store excesses of specific emotions came in 1968 when I began studying acupuncture literature. I was very skeptical but, somehow, my mind remained open to the possibility. (I can't take credit for this openness on a conscious level but somehow it happened.)

Despite my initial skepticism, I have come to accept that the following correspondences exist and are reliable just because they keep showing up in patient after patient since 1968. These internal organ-emotional—we might call them "visceroemotional" correspondences— are as follows:

The Liver

The liver collects, stores and is the seat of anger and depression. The first time I really became convinced of this relationship was when I treated a patient who was at the time an inpatient in a psychiatric ward. She had made three apparently valid but unsuccessful attempts at suicide. She was deep in depression, so deep that speaking was an effort, moving was seldom voluntary, and to be honest about it, I could hardly see her breathe. Her skin color was a yellowish white and transparent. I could feel the hopelessness of this poor woman as soon as she entered my space. She was about 60 years old. She had fallen into this depression about 10 years prior when an air crash killed her son. She was a 20-year divorcee before I met her. She came with her sister who had obtained permission from the psychiatrist for a day pass.

Her liver felt like a bowling ball in both size and consistency. It felt like it weighed about 20 pounds. I put my hands anterior and posterior on her body so that the liver was between them. She was supine on the treatment table. Attempting to release her liver in this way was like trying to dissolve this bowling ball with my hands. I decided to acupuncture for depression according to Felix Mann's recipe as given in his book *Acupuncture, Treatment of Many Diseases*. I put needles in acupuncture points Liver 6, 8 and 13 bilaterally. I went back to her liver with my hands and could feel it begin to soften and respond much more readily to my passage of energy through it. As the liver softened and released, I felt energy forces come from her skin in the front, back and right side where it overlays the liver. Her breathing deepened visibly; her color changed from yellowish white to pinkish white; she began to move a little voluntarily and her face began to show traces of transient expressions. In short, she started looking less like a jaundiced zombie and more like an uncomfortable human who still had some fight left in her. I stayed with the liver until its release seemed complete. I did not dialogue with her, but I kept up a constant patter of encouragement in my mind. Silently, I was urging her to let it go.

After her liver had softened and released the heavy, heavy energy that I assume was her depression, she got a little feisty. She complained about the needles and how long everything was taking. I then went to her craniosacral system and re-leased the compression that was present in the lumbo-sacral junction, the occipital cranial base at the atlas and between the sphenoid, petrous temporals and occiput. When she left, you could hardly tell she was depressed. Mostly, she was angry and complaining about everything.

I saw this woman on two more occasions at weekly intervals. I did additional manual release of the energy of anger from her liver. No further acupuncture was used. I treated the craniosacral system, releasing mostly temporal bone and tentorial membrane restrictions on the next two visits. She was discharged from the hospital after her second visit with me because she had a "spontaneous remission" of her depression. (Her sister did not tell the psychiatrist I was treating her when she took her out on the day passes.) By the third visit, she had stopped taking all her medi-cations. She remained fine for six months after our final session and I have not heard from her or her sister since.

This experience made me consider that, perhaps, a major depressive shock such as the sudden and surprising loss of a son, was absorbed into this woman's liver. Her liver was overwhelmed by the size of the shock. It became a seat of anger at the fates for taking her son from her. It also became a seat of despondency be-cause there was nothing she could do about the death. Since the liver could not handle it all, it then became the ongoing source of the continuing depressive en-ergy and underlying anger that contaminated her whole emotional being. In my mind, I likened the liver to a filter. It might be considered as similar to the oil filter in your car. This filter acts as a cleaner of oil until the filter cartridge is full, then it becomes a source of dirt for the oil in your car's engine. If you change the dirty oil and put in clean oil but do not install a new oil filter, the dirty filter cartridge soon contaminates your new, fresh, clean oil. Perhaps this is what psychotherapy does for depression: It puts in clean oil but if the liver filter isn't cleansed or released, it constantly recontaminates the emotional being with depressive and angry energy. This was a powerful lesson that this generous lady so unselfishly provided. Re-member, every patient you see is an educational opportunity. After this lesson with the liver as a filter, seat and storage bin for anger and depression, I was much more open to the idea that other viscera could filter out and store specific emotions.

The Heart

The heart is the filter, seat and storage bin of the fear of being hurt by loving someone who may not return your love or who may desert you. An injured heart that is protecting itself against the fear of repeating a similar experience will not allow its owner to give unconditional love. The owner of this protecting heart fears entering a true, loving relationship. These owners are afraid of getting hurt again. Some of this fear may be valid, but life without a true love relationship is an empty life indeed. It seems that to really love, we have to trust the person we love. This represents a risk which some people are not willing or able to take. These people may rationally want to love but are emotionally unable to do so.

The offer of conditional love, that is, "I'll love you if you'll love me back," is a sign that the fear in the heart needs to be released—if the patient wants to enter a full and satisfying love relationship. An interesting sign of this fear in the heart that prevents unconditional love is the prenuptial agreement. It seems to say, "I love you, but I'm not sure, and just in case…." Release fear in such a person's heart and they may burn their prenuptial agreement.

Also be aware that unconditional love relationships do not necessarily have to be with a mate or of a sexual nature. It may be with a sibling, a parent, a friend or anyone else. Unconditional love leads to accepting other people's imperfections as well as your own. Once we accept the imperfect state of humanity and have released the fear in our hearts, unconditional love for everyone can follow.

As I'm sure you know by now, I believe that examples and illustrations are very important aids to learning. Therefore, I give you the example of a politician I worked with as a therapeutic facilitator for about three years. This is a female politician. (Certain liberties are taken in describing her case in order to protect her identity.) Originally she began to see me in order to discover why she was 50 pounds overweight and could not lose the weight. The more successful she became, the more weight she gained and the less successful she was at dieting.

A lot of deep work showed several contributing factors to the weight problem. Among them were remembrances as a tiny child of her grandmother who, as a successful national politician, frequently talked in the patient's presence about "throwing your weight around" in order to be a success in politics. She also used to say that one "had to be big enough to cast a shadow that could not be ignored." We also got into the idea that as an adolescent, she decided that the only way to develop an ample bosom (in order to attract male admiration) was to be overweight. When she went on a diet, she lost breast tissue which, deep in her heart, she felt was necessary in order to be an attractive female. The patient was in her mid- and late-40s when I worked with her. She had borne three children with an alcoholic husband. She had divorced several years prior and before she decided to become a professional politician.

All of these insights helped to some extent with the weight problem. She was able to lose and keep off about 25 of the 50 unwanted pounds. Then a romantic episode came into her life. It was the same man for whom she wanted an ample bosom when she was about 14 years of age and he was about 24. She thought she needed breasts to get his attention. She now fell deeply in love with him but discovered that she was very afraid to answer "yes" to his proposal of marriage. She created a multitude of logical reasons to be afraid but she really wanted to love him and be with him. Among her reasons to decline his proposal were the following: He wanted to semi-retire and sail the Caribbean on his yacht. She wanted to keep moving upward with her political aspirations. What if he cheated on her? What if he fell out of love after awhile? What if, what if, what if?

Her heart felt like a piece of stone in a pericardium that was made out of an unsanforized fabric designed for strength and durability which had shrunk and imprisoned the heart. The pericardium is the heart protector and will frequently almost strangle the heart in an attempt to protect it from further injury. I knew that the heart was very fearful of becoming involved in an unconditional love, and the pericardium was certainly doing a great job of insulating this fearful heart.

As we worked with imagery, dialogue and toward manual release of the heart's fear and pericardial overprotection, we came to a vivid memory of a time which covered about the first three days of her post-partum life. She was brought in to be with her mother after she was cleaned and her mother had recovered from the anesthesia. She was put on her mother's breast but nothing came as she suckled. This event recurred several times during the first few days after delivery. Finally, her mother became exasperated and angry with herself—as described by the third-party observer which the patient had become. In her anger, her mother then rejected breastfeeding as a viable method of nurturing her child. The patient took the end of breastfeeding attempts as a personal rejection. She accepted her mother's anger as being a result of something she was or had done.

During the first three days of her life, the patient's pattern was set. She was afraid to love unconditionally because she would be rejected again. After all, she had loved her mother. Her mother got mad at her and wouldn't give her mother's milk. The logic that she developed went something like this: "If you love, people see your faults; then they can leave you or reject you." A solid basis for fear of loving was put into place during the first week of her life.

In addition—and I'm sure you can see it coming—the mother's feelings of breast inadequacy was broadcast into the infant. As our infant grew to adolescence, she was determined not to have the same inadequacies as her mother, so if she had to get fat to get adequate breasts, that is exactly what she would do—and continue to do throughout her life.

Release of the pericardial shielding device and the stone of fear from this lady's heart has impacted her life significantly. She has married the man she loves with only minor trepidation. She has dropped her "what ifs" and seems to be quite happy with him. She has done some cruising with him on his yacht and likes it better than she thought she might. She has gotten out of politics after a few face-saving maneuvers. She seems happy, content and deeply in love for the first time in her life. And she really trusts her husband. She is now vulnerable should her husband turn out to be a cad—but it seems that deep and magnificent rewards require risk. On the other hand, if you believe and trust, there is no risk because you know that all will be taken care of and work out for the best.

The Pericardium

The pericardium is the protector of the heart. When the heart has been hurt, the pericardium springs into action and shields it from further injury. This is a wonderful defense mechanism, but it seems to me that once called into action the pericardium has a very powerful tendency to be overly protective. You cannot release the fear in the heart unless you release the pericardium, either at the same time or beforehand. The example just given clearly illustrates how well the heart

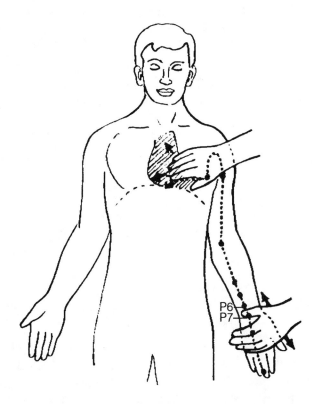

The pericardium (shaded) protects the heart from further pain and the pericardium meridian through which pericardial restriction can be released. See text.
Illustration V–1

and pericardium work in conjunction with each other. I have had hundreds of examples from patients/clients that demonstrate that there cannot be real unconditional love if the pericardium is busy protecting the heart. I frequently use the pericardial meridian as a release valve. The access to this meridian that I most often connect with is on the volar surface of the wrist where the meridian crosses the transverse skin creases of the wrist.

I use this as a "sink" or drain for energy in the pericardium. Place one hand over the pericardium on the left side of the anterior chest. With the other hand, place two or three fingers along the meridian at the wrist between the points designated P6 and P7 on Illustration V-1. Now, imagine energy flowing from the chest to the wrist. (You can, if you wish, cycle it back from the patient's wrist, through your body to the patient's chest, thus completing the loop. Do so if it feels appropriate to you.) If you encounter stiff resistance in the meridian, send the energy back and forth between your hands so that it is going distal for a few seconds then proximal for a few seconds, then distal again and proximal again. Keep doing this until the resistance wears down and the meridian feels open.

Once open, the pericardium can soften and relax. You may have to dialogue with the pericardium and try to convince it that the patient really wants it to relax so that they can experience the joy of unconditional love. You may have to discuss trust, risk, vulnerability and so on. The patient/client may decide (along with the pericardium) to not take the risk. That is the individual's choice. Your responsibility is to enlighten, not force compliance with your views and opinions.

The Lungs

The lungs will serve as a filter, seat and a storage organ for grief. It would seem that the overloading of unresolved grief in the lungs is often the underlying cause for asthma, chronic bronchitis, respiratory allergies, shortness of breath for no apparent reason, and so on. Rib cages won't move right, diaphragms won't allow deep breathing. I also believe that some people use the narcotic effect of tobacco smoke to deaden the pain of the grief in the lungs. (At some point in my career, I would really like to test this hypothesis.)

There are numerous cases in our files that illustrate the release of grief from the lungs. This grief is identified as it passes through conscious awareness upon its release. An interesting patient that I had the privilege of working with was a woman in her early 30s. She had developed asthma following the C-section delivery of an eight-month fetus who lived only a few hours. She kept a stiff upper lip because she did not want to emotionally injure her other children who were two and five years of age. She developed respiratory problems shortly after the delivery. She was diagnosed as asthmatic.

Craniosacral evaluation with arcing, fascial glide and symmetry of craniosacral motion gave the impression that the fascias of her thorax were not moving, but there was no active lesion pathology. The dural tube was restricted from the lower cervical region to the thoracolumbar junction. When I placed my hands on her thorax, it felt like it was full of cement. It felt heavy like grief. Using SomatoEmotional Release, Therapeutic Imagery and Dialogue, we established the need to complete the delivery vaginally and to complete the grieving process—both in the lung tissues and emotionally. This was done and the asthma left as quickly as it came.

The Kidneys

The kidneys are often the filter, seat and storage organs for another kind of fear. I call this fear, either correctly or incorrectly, the fear of mortality. By this, I mean the fear that when you die, it's all over; there is no progeny to continue the chromosomal lineage. One might philosophize that in order for the species to continue each individual is embodied with an instinct to reproduce and thus achieve a sort of chromosomal immortality. Fear that you will not reproduce and thus continue your genetic lineage is filtered and stored in the kidneys.

This kind of problem is present in many men as they contemplate vasectomy and in women who are considering tubal ligation or hysterectomy. It can be seen in parents awaiting grandparenthood if the process seems to be taking too long. It shows up in parents who endure the death of a child who has not yet reproduced. Women who have had miscarriages or abortions and have no living children will often demonstrate fear in the kidneys. This fear should be released from the kidneys. It will frequently require confrontation with the reality that there may be no progeny for any number of reasons.

Release of the fear usually is not too difficult but your skills may well be taxed as you try to bring about acceptance of the situation as it is. That patient's chromosomal future often has its end in sight and this is not easily accepted. Recognition of the underlying problem is mandatory. Acceptance and resolution are also necessary or the kidneys will refill with fear.

The fear-filled kidney shows itself as sexual dysfunction, recurrent bladder infections or inflammations, chronic anxiety, perfectionism and high blood pressure. A 65-year-old man that I worked with for several years suffered from chronic kidney dysfunction manifested by blood, albumen and uric acid crystals in the urine. He also suffered from severe heart disease—both valvular (aortic and ventral) and arterial—and from severe hypertension. He ultimately died of heart failure.

His course illustrates the role of fear in the kidneys and the effect on his total physiology. I was not able to get an acceptance and resolution of the cause of the fear. His fear was well founded. He was 65 and had never sired a child. As far as he was concerned, when he died his chromosomal or genetic lineage ended. He could not accept an eternal soul concept as a viable alternative. He really wanted his genes to be passed along.

The point of the case is that we were able to empty the fear from his kidneys periodically using SomatoEmotional Release and Therapeutic Imagery and Dialogue. He had weekly urine studies and daily blood pressure readings. He was well monitored by internal medicine specialists in heart and kidney function. When his kidneys felt void of the cold, heavy energy that I am calling fear, his urinalysis studies moved toward normal, his cardiac function improved and his blood pressure normalized. These changes would last for two to three weeks, then his test results and function would regress to abnormal again. We worked together over a period of five years and observed this roller coaster effect probably 10 times a year.

Each time we discharged the fear, he rallied significantly but we could never get past the idea that when he died his whole ancestral lineage went with him. He was an only child and felt the burden of responsibility to carry on his family name and the family genes. His parents had placed this burden on his shoulders very early in his life. So not only was death scary, it was failure. The poor man died following a cardiac catherization test that a new cardiologist convinced him he needed.

All cases are not so dreary, but recognize that you may have to do a powerful lot of talking and convincing to get the barren patient past the fear that strikes when the end of their chromosomal lineage is in sight. If the outlook is not so bleak, you may be able to help them see that all they need is a child or a grandchild to keep their kidneys clear of this kind of fear of mortality.

The Spleen

The spleen filters and stores the disappointment of the type that results from observation of man's inhumanity to man. (Sorry about the sexist use of the male gender in this quote, but that is how it is said. Better yet, perhaps women are not inhumane.) Probably the best example that I can give of this type of splenic disappointment is my own rather dramatic experience with such a release. I was being treated by an Advanced CranioSacral Therapy class. In short order, attention was quickly focused upon my spleen. Soon I visualized a hollow bamboo tube coming straight up and out of my spleen. Then a yellow liquid began issuing forth through the bamboo tube and onto the floor. As this occurred—and it seemed to last for an hour—I felt a sensation of my spleen deflating.

During this time of extrusion of the yellow liquid of disappointment from my spleen, I imaged a newsreel of the wars and atrocities that we humans do to one another: I saw Israelis and Arabs killing each other; I saw bombings and warlike activity in Northern Ireland; I saw the Falkland Islands war between Britain and Argentina; I saw us in Vietnam and I saw the Crusaders killing people in the name of God.

Before this treatment I could become livid with anger when I thought about our social injustices, unnecessary killing and massacres. I considered these things as unforgivable and could almost give myself a stroke or heart attack just thinking about them. After the release of the energy of disappointment from the spleen, I still feel badly about what we humans do to each other but am not so affected physiologically or emotionally by things I cannot immediately affect. I will still work against them but the tremendous emotional upset does not accompany the knowledge. Now I simply accept that people have a lot more evolving to do before they will treat each other humanely. And now I also know that people will never do what I want them to do, so I'm not so disappointed when they don't follow my rules.

With patients, I dialogue routinely with all of the emotions in the various organs. I ask them about their origins, how they feel about things today and what they would like for tomorrow. I ask if they would like to convert to something less demanding or consuming on the host's physiological resources. I try to work out as nice a resolution as possible with the organ that is saturated or filled to capacity with a particular emotion. My advice to you is to explore—and don't be surprised by anything that occurs.

A MODEL FOR THE PATIENT-FACILITATOR CONNECTION

It seems to be really helpful to have a model from which you can work when you are exploring. I learned some of the value of modeling in a very practical way when Dr. Zvi Karni (a biophysicist) and I developed the PressureStat model to explain the craniosacral system.

We are now presented with the question of what happens when a bodyworker turned CranioSacral Therapist turned holistic therapeutic facilitator works with a patient. The model I have developed is quite simple. (It can be shown to have defects, but it does help answer questions about what is going on in the therapeutic-facilitative session and so it serves a purpose. It also raises questions, creates controversy and will hopefully stimulate further creative thought. In so doing it serves yet another important purpose. I will defend this model partly to provoke thought and partly because it works. I have little or no actual investment of pride or ego in it.)

The model looks like Illustration V-2. I am optimistic that we will all agree that the goal of the therapeutic-facilitative process is the development of a nice, easy, flowing line of communication and connectedness between the patient's con-

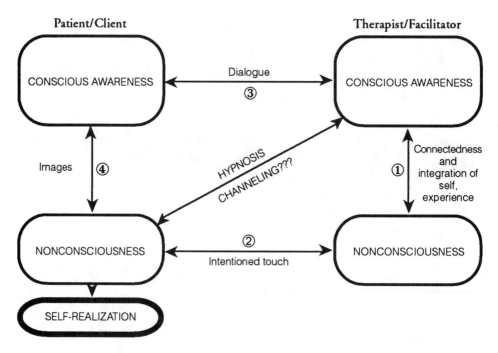

Model steps in connecting patient with achieving self-realization, the goal of therapy.
Illustration V–2

scious awareness and his/her nonconscious. (I use the word nonconscious rather than unconscious because I want to cut across the limiting boundaries of the various schools of psychology. I want to avoid the baggage that the word "unconscious" has accumulated.) The nonconscious, for our present purposes, refers to anything not readily accessible to our conscious awareness upon unassisted first or second request. The nonconscious refers to any part of us—from the highest self to the lowest subconscious of which we are unaware. The term "nonconscious" avoids the hierarchy that so many psychospiritual models foster.

The skills and abilities of a therapeutic facilitator depend largely upon openness of communication between his/her own conscious awareness and nonconscious. That is, how readily does nonconscious information come into the conscious awareness of the therapeutic facilitator? Further, how readily is the conscious intent of the therapeutic facilitator transmitted to, received by and acted upon by his/her own nonconscious? Ultimately, there is a blending and an openness of communication between the various levels of consciousness and the hands, the total body, the emotions, the spirit and the awareness of this therapeutic facilitator.

This connectedness is represented by the dually-directed arrow numbered 1 in Illustration V-2. This connectedness may—and probably will—change during the session, but it does preexist. For most bodyworkers or hands-on people, the first touch represents the first meaningful encounter with the patient/client.

Intentioned touch is labeled number 2 in Illustration V-2 because the accomplished therapeutic facilitator usually has number 1 in place before he or she enters the therapeutic facilitation session. Some therapeutic facilitators do gain much information from the first look at the patient and the exchange of amenities. But let us say that the work really begins when the first intentioned touch occurs. (Number 2 in our model.)

"Intentioned" means that the therapeutic facilitator has either consciously or nonconsciously given instructions to herself/himself that the session has begun and "Let's get to work." The information comes flooding into the nonconscious from his/her hands. Some or all of the input is routed into the therapeutic facilitator's conscious awareness for consideration. Intentioned touch also means that the message to the patient from the therapeutic facilitator is, "I'm here to help. I won't judge. I'll try to provide generic energy—no strings attached—compassion, strength, courage and whatever you sincerely need, including unlimited and unconditional love as you sincerely need it." In short, you, as the therapeutic facilitator, are there for the patients/clients. Your hands tell them so.

This two-way exchange of information begins between your two nonconsciousnesses almost immediately with the first intentioned touch. Hence your attitude has an immediate impact on the patient/client's nonconscious. Be sure that your head is in the right space to therapeutically facilitate. If it isn't, you may facilitate the establishment of defenses that can be very difficult to overcome later.

If your own nonconscious communication lines with your conscious awareness are open, you will immediately begin to receive information from the patient/client's nonconscious into his/her nonconscious and from there into your conscious awareness. You must also be aware of your attitude and should modify that attitude in order to give comfort and confidence to the patient/client in a nonconscious way.

You may also program your patients/clients for healing. They need not be aware of it. You can feel their fear, their resentment, their guilt, their anger, their joy and their optimism through your touch and your open nonconscious-conscious communication lines. (You need not speak a word or you can discuss the weather, a basketball game, a recent movie or whatever.) This evaluative process is not simply feeling body tissue tension. It is literally sensing the nonconscious emotional makeup of the patient by the use of connecting touch. You can also sense physical feelings and memories through connecting touch. Actually, there seems to be no limit as you continue to open communication lines between your conscious awareness and your nonconsciousness.

In our working model (Illustration V-2) number 3 represents the opening of meaningful verbal communication between the conscious awareness of the patient and that of the therapeutic facilitator. Correctly used, the Significance Detector[19] will indicate which subjects represent the most fertile ground for further work.

As we touch and talk, we begin to reach with our hands through our patient/clients' nonconsciousness toward their conscious awareness. At the same time, our words begin to reach through their conscious awareness into their nonconsciousness. Thus, we begin the connectedness work from both ends, creating overlap so that number 4 in the model (Illustration V-2) begins to establish itself.

As the work progresses, working together we will usually be able to elicit images from the patient/client's nonconscious. Next, we can discuss the images as they come forth. Soon we can dialogue with the images directly. As this dialogue is established, be aware that you are privileged, as a therapeutic facilitator, to be conversing with some level or part of the patient/client's nonconscious. As the ease of dialogue with images progresses, the goal of therapeutic facilitation comes closer and closer. Patients/clients begin to gain insights into and about themselves. They also begin to realize their potential for self-healing.

Sometimes it may occur that the communication goes directly from the nonconscious of the patient/client to the conscious awareness of the therapeutic facilitator. This occurrence looks a lot like deep hypnosis, and probably is (although

[19] The Significance Detector is the sudden cessation of the craniosacral rhythm. It can be used to tell the practitioner whether or not a word, thought or body position is significant. Also see *CranioSacral Therapy II, Beyond the Dura*, p. 216.

it may also look like channeling at times). In either case, it seems to occur when the nonconscious (in the case of deep relaxation) or the guide (in the case of channeling) does not feel that the patient/client is ready to recognize the information being offered. When this appears to be the case, I always instruct patients as they return to the here and now that they can remember or not remember what has occurred during the session. It is their choice.

I also discuss with the nonconscious spokesperson or guide his/her particular preference about how much I should tell the patient after he/she comes out of the deep relaxation state. I do feel that it is ultimately (almost always) necessary that the content of the session be brought into the patient/client's conscious awareness. I will discuss this opinion with the nonconscious spokesperson or the guide. I try to point out the benefit of bringing this content and the insights that can follow into the conscious awareness. I like to make it a question of "when" not "if." Once this is accomplished, I gently try to work the acceptable time of disclosure closer to the present.

Don't push too hard. I have had two lessons from patients that illustrate the importance of conscious unreadiness and conscious readiness for the content presented by the nonconscious. I should like to share these two experiences with you at this time.

TIMING

First, let's consider the case of a young man who came to my office in 1965. He came in because he wanted to use hypnosis for weight reduction. I had been on a medical panel which was broadcast by a local television station, and during the show, we had discussed various uses of hypnosis in anesthesia, as a behavior modifier and as a means of accessing suppressed information, memories, feelings and experiences. This 24-year-old man named Michael had seen the show. He was five feet, 10 inches tall and weighed 320 pounds. He stated that he had weighed over 200 pounds in the eighth grade, and his eating and drinking of high calorie sodas had been out of control for as long as he could remember. He had tried almost every diet he had ever heard of and never lasted more than five to 10 days on any of them. Appetite suppressant pills, legal in those days, made him so nervous that he could not use them. Michael was very ready to try hypnoregression to search for the psycho-emotional reasons for his uncontrollable abuse of food and soft drinks. (He denied the use of alcohol.)

Michael was an excellent hypnotic subject and was induced into a deep trance during the first session. While in the trance, I had him discuss with me the reasons that he wanted to lose weight. He told me that he used his weight as a protection against being hurt. I asked him if he was willing to look for the reasons he needed the fat shield and if he would share those reasons with me. Michael's nonconscious agreed and we began the regression.

I first asked Michael to go back to a happy time, before he was fat. He went back to the fourth grade where he was on the stage and in the school spelling bee contest. He recalled the words and spelled them for me. He described the girl left in the contest competing against him. Then he described her erroneous spelling of her word and how sorry he felt for her. But the sympathy was short lived, as he spelled the word correctly. He won! It felt wonderful!

Then it felt awful. The teacher in charge disqualified Michael because he had words that were used in the spelling bee written on a tiny paper that he took from his pocket after he had won the bee. He was accused of cheating. He denied that he had looked at the paper while he spelled his words, that the paper was how he studied. His appeals were to no avail, and he was disqualified from the spelling bee.

He went to his grandmother's house after school because he was ashamed to face his mother. Grandma believed him. She fed him milk and cookies and cake and ice cream. She told him not to worry, she would protect him. Somehow, he connected the food administered by Grandma with his protection against the world and failures and accusations. He began to eat for protection on that day and had been compulsively putting away excess calories ever since.

I brought Michael out of the trance slowly. As I did so, I instructed him that the next time we met he would go deeply into the special sleep where we could talk to his unconscious again. (I was saying "unnconscious" in those days.) I also suggested that he would feel fine and rested when he awoke. I further let him know that he would remember only that which he could handle or deal with when he awoke. Anything that was too much for him he could leave in his nonconscious for the time being. Michael remembered nothing when he awoke. He felt fine. He asked a few innocuous questions and left the office.

He had three more weekly appointments, all of which were much the same as the first. We continued to identify the spelling bee episode as the initial cause for his need for protection and his grandmother as the factor that started him using calories and the resulting fat as the preferred protection against the cruel world in which we live. (I was not experienced and knowledgeable enough at the time to use desensitizing techniques, the other more subtle approaches to help Michael deal with the problem.) After each of the four weekly sessions, he had no recall of the content of the session. He asked a few questions, but it was obvious that he really didn't seem to want to know much about what had happened. I did not know how to prepare him for the insight that I felt would be a major step forward in his treatment.

At the end of the fifth session, he again let me know that he had no recall of what had happened. I told him about the spelling bee, his grandma and the eating for comfort and fat for protection. He didn't believe me. We discussed it some more. In just a few minutes he panicked and ran (waddled rapidly) from the office. He never came back and I never heard from Michael again.

I really blew that one. This incident is a good example of how not to help your patient confront reality. I was insensitive to his needs and fears. (I hadn't even thought about such a thing as a craniosacral system as yet.) I was in the business of "fixing" people. I sure fixed Michael. I do thank him if he is out there somewhere because I have never forgotten the lesson he gave me. This lesson gains meaning with each year that passes in my life as a therapeutic facilitator. Now I appreciate much more fully the work it may take to move from an unready to a ready conscious awareness.

Now, let's consider another educational experience that a patient was kind enough to give me. This second example describes what can happen when the timing is right and conscious awareness is ready for a major piece of insight and self-awareness.

Reta was 38 years old when she came to see me. The year was 1966. I was still pondering what had happened to Michael. He seemed to have disappeared. I had vowed never to be insensitive and overly forceful about reality confrontation again. Reta was the mother of four children, all still in school. She was the wife of an engineer who sometimes worked and sometimes didn't. She was the very valued, efficient and underpaid executive secretary of a local bank president.

Reta was referred to me because she had uncontrollable and unremitting pain in the head, neck, upper thorax, shoulders, arms and hands. She had less frequent but episodically severe low back and right sciatic pain. She was referred by an orthopedic surgeon who couldn't find anything else to cut on. He had operated on her three times already. He had been unsuccessful in helping her. I had developed some small reputation as a pain controller who used hypnosis, trigger-injection, manipulation and whatever else was available. I also did a pretty fair brand of general medicine and minor surgery. Reta was probably a nuisance to the orthopod by now, as well as a reminder that he had failed. He knew that I would take the night calls because I was young and eager and rather taken with myself.

Reta had been surgically cut up and generally punished by life significantly. She had her varicose veins surgically removed. She had a hysterectomy after her fourth obstetrical delivery. All four children had been delivered vaginally with wide episiotomies. She then underwent a repair of the perineum and a bladder suspension (both done before the hysterectomy). She then had her gallbladder removed. This referring orthopedic surgeon had removed discs from between the third and fourth as well as from between the fourth and fifth lumbar vertebrae. These were done on two separate occasions. After this, he had unsuccessfully attempted nerve root decompression in the lower cervical region.

In addition to all of this, her children were very demanding of her time and energy. They offered very little respect. Her husband was physically abusive of her episodically. He was psycho-emotionally abusive of her all the time. Her boss always asked for a little more than she could do.

Today this history would have told me the story of a need for self-punishment. Back then, I just felt sorry for her. I simply listened to her story, examined her body, felt a lot of compassion and vowed aloud that we would get to the bottom of this problem. Reta and I made a pact that we would both give it our best and go wherever the trail led us. (This was very unprofessional behavior in those days). I would see her twice weekly.

I began with trigger injection and manipulation. The first treatment produced relief for a few days. When the pain came back it had changed its distribution somewhat and was a little worse in severity. To make a long story short, about 10 trigger injection and manipulation sessions got us nowhere. I recall the last trigger injection session we had. The pain kept moving from one place to another around her upper back, thorax, neck, shoulders, arms and hands as I injected and manipulated. It was as though the pain were running away from my trigger injections. That night I injected 18 triggers. This was a record for me, but we were determined to win.

Needless to say, we did not win with that approach. Reta's pain got much worse after that session. Hit by the sledgehammer of failure, I realized that trigger injections were not the way to fly. I thought I had better think a little about what to do next. Meanwhile, Reta was unable to sleep because of her pain. I suggested that she try to learn some self-hypnosis so that she could at least lessen the pain and get some sleep.

After a few sessions (during which I attempted to teach her how to hypnotize herself to sleep), she spontaneously went into a deep trance. This would suggest to me today that her nonconscious had checked me out and decided that I wasn't the best but was at least sincere and better than nothing. I was suddenly inspired to search for the cause of the pain using hypnoregression. Almost immediately, Reta regressed to memories of age five, age four, age three, age two and age one. She lost her ability to converse as she got younger and younger and preverbal in her development. I suggested that her right hand would be able to write the answers to my questions as an adult, no matter how little she was during her experience. Lo and behold, she could do it. At age one she indicated that the reason for her pain had already been put into place. She just wrote this information down for me on a stenographer's notepad with her adult right hand.

I asked her to go back to the time when the reason for the pain was implanted. This was a tedious process because she could not talk intelligibly to me so she had to write everything out for me. I didn't know at that time that I could have a "witness" part of her go up on the ceiling and describe the scene to me. After many questions and a lot of slowly written answers (people write rather slowly under these circumstances), Reta regressed to age two days. She had been born at home and was lying in a cradle. Her mother and maternal grandmother were there. Her grandmother was admonishing her mother for having had another baby at her age. The mother was 42 at the time of Reta's birth, and Reta was the youngest of eight children. Grandma said that, "Reta should never had been born. It was too hard on [the mother]." Grandma also said that Reta would never be healthy.

The imposition of guilt and hopelessness brought upon Reta by this conversation was phenomenal. I shall never forget what Reta wrote when I asked her how she felt about this scene: "If I had to be born, if I had to live, at least I can be weak, sick and hurt all my life."

When Reta came out of her regressed state, I very gently asked her if she could read what was written on the paper. She could not. She asked if I could read it, and I pretended I could not. She accepted my explanation without question because she wanted to believe me.

Three days later we repeated the same regression to the cradle, and she listened to her grandmother talking to her mother. She wrote me the same statement again about how she felt. This time, I was a little wiser. I told her that the pregnancy had not been instigated by her. I told her that all had gone well. Her mother had survived the delivery without difficulty. I told her that her grandmother probably meant well but that her observations were not correct. I wasn't sure I'd gotten through to her because Reta was still the two-day-old infant when I delivered my speech. Again, I let her know as she returned to the here and now that she did not need to comprehend anything she was not ready for. I was painstakingly careful about imparting the message to her. (I remembered Michael very clearly.) She could not read her handwritten message.

Four days later, Reta came in again. Trance was quickly induced. I asked her to go to the experience whereby she became convinced that she could not be without pain. She went straight to the same cradle scene. She heard her grandmother's words to her mother for the third time. I delivered my lecture again about the pregnancy not being Reta's responsibility and so on. Then, I intuitively brought her back to adulthood while she was still in deep trance. We discussed the situation while in trance as an adult. Reta agreed that it was not valid that she should spend her life in pain because of her grandmother's emotional words to her mother. We also agreed that she would be able to handle the insight after she came out of trance. I brought Reta back to her usual state of conscious awareness. She was able to read her notes. (There were three sets of them now.) She simply asked whether she could have done all of this to herself. I replied that it seemed reasonable.

Strange as it seems, that was the end of Reta's pain. She divorced her husband. She quit her job and started her own real estate company in partnership with a man who eventually became her husband.

Reta was an excellent teacher for me. I am forever grateful to her. In retrospect, Reta's case suggests that our nonconsciouses were definitely connected before my own conscious awareness was well connected to my own nonconscious. Why do I say this? There are several clues. Her pain got worse when I was doing the trigger injections. We made a pact to follow through to successful completion no matter what. (I never did things like that.) Intuitively, I used hypnosis for sleep and pain control. Reta took it to hypnoregression. I was in way over my head trying to work with a two-day-old infant back in 1966. I had no idea what to do, but looking back it feels like Reta's nonconscious told mine what to do. Then I just did what my intuition told me to do without much forethought or question. Looks like a setup to me.

If I had gone easier with Michael or changed my timing, he might have come to grips with the cause of his obesity. As it is, I did him no favor. I only pray that he connected with his nonconscious at a later date and was able to handle what came up. With Reta, I listened more carefully—although I wasn't aware that I was listening. It worked out wonderfully well. Timing and sensitivity are critical. That which is unacceptable now might work fine an hour from now.

One other point about timing that bears repeating: You should always get the patient/client to make the discoveries, no matter how much time it takes to get to this. Don't just blurt out what is abundantly clear to you about the situation. Help patients/clients to discover, but don't tell the answer. Make them thirsty. Show them the water, but they have to do their own drinking.

ATTITUDES

We have spoken a little about attitudes previously, but before we go on to the next subject I want to make it crystal clear that there is no doubt left in my mind that the attitudes of both the patient/client and the therapeutic facilitator very strongly influence the outcome of the therapeutic session. The nonconscious connection makes the attitude of the patient/client accessible to you as the therapeutic facilitator just as your attitude is accessible to the patient/client.

Do not ever forget this fact. Do not think you can fake a positive attitude when you don't have one. The attitudinal impressions that come into the nonconscious of one of us from the other during a session may or may not surface into conscious awareness. The negative attitude may simply produce a sense of uneasiness or distrust that is sort of indefinable. It may produce a dislike of the other for no apparent reason or it may produce a sense of futility. It may even produce a feeling of impatience to get out of the same space from the other.

When you, as the therapeutic facilitator, sense something that may be of attitudinal origin and it seems capable of interfering with a good joint effort between you and the patient/client, you must decide whether it is an attitude in yourself that is making itself known or whether it is coming from the patient/client. This determination should not present much of a problem. Consider that your intentioned touch has opened communication lines that go both ways between the nonconscious of both the patient/client and you. If you use a little mental energy, you can construct a barrier of your choosing between the two of you. You can stop all communication in both directions. You can exclusively stop your input into the patient/client or you can exclusively stop patient/client input. In addition, you can stop patient/client input at any selected region of your body and can selectively allow only certain energies to enter you from the patient/client. With all of these tools and techniques available to you, it takes just a little creative manipulation of energies to discover the source (or sources) of the obstructive/destructive attitude. If you block input from the patient/client and the attitude disappears, it is most likely that the patient/client owns it. If you stop all of your output into the patient/client and the attitude persists, it is probably yours and it must come into your conscious awareness to let you know. If, when you interrupt all communication between the two of you, the attitude disappears, it is probably the patient/client's property; if it stays it is yours.

What do you do when you discover that your attitude presents an obstacle to a good productive therapeutic session? The best choice, of course, is to change your attitude now that you are aware of it. It may or may not have something to do with this patient/client. It may just be a piece of your own baggage that you neglected to leave at the door of the treatment room. You can usually just focus and clear yourself and eliminate this piece of undesirable baggage from the session. It may be that the patient/client's appearance, conduct, energy or whatever stirs a memory in you that is not altogether a pleasant one. In this case, recognize it and try to divorce the patient/client from the memory. The main thing is recognition.

Whatever the reason for the attitudinal problem, you can choose to terminate the session because you are not fit to work at that time. This, however, is a very impractical approach. A few premature terminations of treatment sessions can give the impression that you are a self-indulgent, undisciplined, spoiled and immature brat. This word can go out on the grapevine and devastate a practice rather quickly.

Instead of ending the session prematurely, I suggest that you excuse yourself for a moment, perhaps leave the room, get yourself focused, centered and cleansed of destructive feelings. Then go back in and start all over. If this does not work and you continue to feel your attitude is an obstacle, work on a more superficial level. Work with more gross structure. Intention your touch not to act as a nonconscious communication line between you. It may occur as you do this that you feel your own attitude shift and you can begin to work more deeply without dumping your stuff on (or into) the patient/client. Remember all things are constantly changing. The therapeutic facilitative endeavor is very dynamic, so it behooves you to continually test the waters.

If you determine that the patient/client owns the obstructive or destructive attitude that you feel, try to consider it as part of the problem which brought them to you in the first place. This does not mean that I believe I can handle any kind of attitude from any patient/client. It means that I will try to consider the attitude as something that will change as the therapeutically facilitative healing process progresses. It may be too much for me. I might get an angry response or a guilt response every time I enter the patient/client's presence. If this happens and I can't control it or rid myself of the reaction, it is time to recognize my own limitations. I should refer the patient/client to someone else and do some work on my own boundaries so that the next time I may not have the same limit.

Yet another consideration is well worth mentioning. In recent conversation with a physicist, he put forth the idea that each of us has at least 50 different energy fields in which we live. He suggests that we generate or modify these energy fields to our needs and our likes. He further suggests that the energy fields of individuals may either attract or repel one another. If this is so, the possibility exists that the best healers are those with the most widely attractive and narrowly repelling energy fields—so that the greater percentage of people are attracted to them. It is not far out of reach to hypothesize that you may meet the occasional patient/client whose energy field is repelled by yours or vice versa.

Can you change your energy field by the use of your mental efforts? Perhaps you can. I think so. Perhaps there are degrees of change. Perhaps some repulsion can be overcome. Some may be so strong as to require too much constant output of will to maintain compatibility.

In addition to the sense of attitude that we have discussed, there is also your attitude toward patients/clients and what they do with images, dialogue and so on that must be kept in mind. Always be grateful, kind, generous, humble, patient and gentle, but be firm and supportive. Subordinate your ego. It doesn't matter what the patient/client images, it is valid. It doesn't matter what you know, let patients/clients discover it. You can plant clues and encourage, but you forfeit a great deal if you tell them the answers rather than help them discover it themselves.

If you feel compelled to tell them the answers to their problems, you had better do some work on your own ego. It is probably because you just have to let them know how smart you are or because you are self-focused and impatient. Cool out and let them explore. Be with them. Be impressed by their insights, even though you think you had the answer two weeks ago. Remember it is the patient/client's session, not yours.

RESISTANCE

Resistance to therapeutic facilitation comes in many forms. It can be very deceptive, yet it seems to me that we can usually assign resistance to one of three major categories:

Suppressed Imagination

Most of us learn to consider our imaginings and fantasies as silly. Although they might be fun, we certainly are not to take them seriously. We also learn that if we talk to ourselves, we are crazy. If we let the wrong people (like doctors) know that we talk to ourselves, we could be put away. If we want to make something of ourselves, we can't be daydreaming, seeing imagined friends, talking to them and so on.

All this negative input about the imagination must be overcome. If you consider all this, it is a miracle that even 10 percent of our patient/clients can image and dialogue productively. Think about it. We, as therapeutic facilitators, can be associated with the same doctors who can put away the patient who talks to himself/herself. We, as teachers, may be connected to the very teachers who told us that we had better stop daydreaming and get down to business if we want to "amount to anything."

Now we sit here touching patients/clients and trying to convince them that an Inner Physician is inside them who they can image as a person and who will talk to them and effectively tell them why they have sciatica or cancer or whatever. Even more ridiculous, this person can tell them how to rid themselves of the problem. How quickly do you suppose you can overcome a lifetime of exposure that dogmatically says what we are doing is ridiculous? It takes recurrent exposures, support and practice to overcome these negative teachings, so don't be impatient. And if you don't believe it yourself, your patient/client may sense your lack of belief and have difficulty doing the work.

Suppression to Avoid Confrontation

We base another category of resistance on suppression of unwanted material. There is often a part of the patient/client's nonconsciousness that protects the patient/client's conscious awareness from an unpleasant confrontation with the suppressed material. The protecting part is working hard to spare the patient/client. The protector is frequently unaware of the symptoms or dysfunctions that relate to the suppressed material. The symptoms or dysfunctions may be the cost of suppression, or they may be an attempt to get attention by another nonconscious part that wants to get this problem solved. In either case, the protector will throw up obstacles and resistance to therapeutic facilitation aiming at increased self-knowledge and awareness.

You must identify the protector and the part that wants the problem identified and resolved. After you identify these characters, you must get to know them and develop a friendly relationship with both of them. Search for their common ground. Discuss the methods both parts are using and how the methods are working antagonistically to each other. Elicit suggestions from both the protector and the part that wants the problem to be resolved, negotiate compromise potential and identify areas of agreement. Try to get the suppressed material out into the open with the agreement of the protector. Then go for a plan that will lead to resolution.

Occasionally, I have encountered a protector who was so tired and so bored with its tedious work that it created symptoms to get attention to request a change of duty, a rest or a little fun. This condition is the exception, but keep your mind open to the possibility and work with it as you find it.

"Contrary" Electrons

The third category of resistance origins requires a little more imagination than the other two. It is a fun idea to play with and if you do play with it, you will most likely expand your limits.

We talked earlier about the possibility that contrary electrons exist. This idea comes forth from the observation that most electrons will perform according to expectation. But there always seem to be a few electrons that behave in the opposite way from that which we expect. We might think of these as "contrary" electrons.

If one chooses to ponder the concept of holographic theory, a sun could be considered a nucleus and the planets its electrons. If there are contrary electrons, there could be contrary planets. If a conscious awareness is comparable to a nucleus, then the various parts of the nonconscious might be considered analogous to the electrons. There then could be naturally contrary parts of the nonconsciousness. Resistance as we see it could be offered by these contrary nonconscious parts.

How Do We Deal With Resistance?

What do we do about resistance? Unequivocally, my highest priority first rule is to treat it with respect. Resistances are not to be overpowered. Resistances are to be enlisted in the process toward healing and growth.

The first category of resistance can usually be overcome by assurance and support. The patient/client may need to read and hear of the successes of other patients/clients who have or are using therapeutic imagery, dialogue, SomatoEmotional Release and the clearing of facilitated segments. Sometimes reading books such as *I Choose Life* or *Love, Medicine and Miracles* is enough. Sometimes it helps to describe to patients/clients other experiences in your practice. Sometimes I ask a patient/client who has successfully healed a tumor, disease or symptom using these techniques to converse with the resistant patient/client.

Most often, a few positive experiences will overcome this kind of resistance.

Ask patients/clients to pretend that anything is possible and—just for now—go with their imagination. If you can get a little bit of physiological or experiential confirmation, it will help to show the power the imagination holds over the body. Get resistant patients/clients to warm their hands by imagining that they are lying in the sun. Or get their mouths to water by imagining one of their favorite foods. The possibilities are infinite. Use your imagination.

I recently worked with a young man who is a chiropractor. He had become a chiropractor largely because he had chronic, unrelenting low back and left leg pain in the sciatic distribution. He had all the adjustments he could handle but the symptoms continued. I helped him to develop his concept of an Inner Physician who was wise and knew all about his health and his body.

We then developed a persona for this Inner Physician by requesting that he please come forward and get acquainted with us. We really wanted to talk with him. We really needed his help. The Inner Physician presented as a wise man who gave out a kindly feeling. He said he understood the back and leg pain as well as its reason for existence. After much dialogue and rapport development, the Inner Physician agreed to show us the reason for the pain.

The patient re-experienced, with some difficulty, standing next to the bed as his older brother died of leukemia at home. He was three years old at the time. After strengthening the communication between nonconscious and conscious awareness, he could hear his aunt tell his mother, right after his brother took his last breath, that at least his brother wouldn't have any more pain. The patient's three-year-old mind interpreted this to mean that if you had pain, you lived. He knew that his brother had experienced a lot of pain the last few months before dying. If you didn't have pain you would die.

So, the nonconscious part of this patient—that made the interpretation that pain was a vital part of life—took on the job of making him hurt every day. It wasn't a pleasant task but it seemed necessary. All we had to do was convince this part of the patient's nonconscious that life would go on and would be of better quality if the pain stopped. The pain did stop and has not recurred since this realization occurred.

The secondary structural corrections were made. Prior to the patient gaining insight into the purpose of the pain, he did not respond to structural correction. Now he responded very well. Still, it took much patience and work to get the cooperation of the Inner Physician on so deep and serious a matter.

The resistance to letting go of the pain was well justified because it felt that it was prolonging the patient's life each day that he hurt. It is fascinating to note that this patient, after understanding his situation, remarked that every morning the first thing he did was check to see if the pain was still there.

We would certainly not have wanted to overpower the patient's resistance if the "pain preserves life" belief had continued. If we had managed to get rid of the pain without resolving its need to be there, it would not have surprised me to see this patient die or at least suffer a life-threatening illness or accident. Identify the resistance, get acquainted, get friendly and understand the reason for the "resistance existence." (I got that from Jessie Jackson.) Then negotiate and reason with the resistance. Assume that the resistance intentions are good.

When you question your patient/client, don't invite a "no" answer. Don't say, "Can you see your Inner Physician?" Instead ask, "How can we get acquainted with your Inner Physician?" With the second question, there is no easy negative answer. The patient doesn't have to visualize to satisfy you. You have taken a positive approach with the tacit assumption that you and the patient/client will get acquainted with the Inner Physician. It isn't "if," it is "when and how" can you, as a therapeutic facilitator, help this to happen.

If an image occurs that is fearful, allow the patient/client to view it from a distance. Suggest that the patient/client imagines that he/she has binoculars or a telescope to see the details of the scary image. As the details are seen and described, you help the patient/client to desensitize the image and, concurrently, what the image represents. For example, as the fear of a fire-blowing dragon is diminished by getting used to it and understanding its details, so will the suppressed childhood memory and fear of a terrible bully who used to terrorize the patient/client also lose some of its potency. It too will become more approachable. You also can ask patients/clients to fly closer to the fearful image. Sometimes it helps to imagine themselves as invisible, so they are totally safe as they approach the threatening image.

You, as the therapeutic facilitator, may offer to be there with the patients/clients as they decide whether to confront a terrifying image or memory. I always do this. Most patients think of me as a powerful person. I use my image to help them. I offer to be there holding their hands in their image of themselves. I offer to share my courage, strength and expertise in the management of such matters. I suggest that together we can do it. This usually works.

If things get too difficult, as in the memory of a rape or abuse, and the protective resistance threatens to interrupt the re-experiencing of an event, I ask patients/clients to try to leave their body. If they can, I have them go up on the ceiling, look down and describe what they see. If this doesn't work, you can have them pretend they are watching a movie. If a movie screen is too large and engulfing, use a television screen. A color movie is more scary than black and white. If a movie screen is too large and engulfing, use a television screen either in color or black and white.

Your goal is to desensitize, using these techniques, so that patients/clients can go through the total experience as participants. Help them overcome fear and protective resistance, but do it gently. Be sensitive to proper timing.

Another resistance that I see often is exemplified by patients/clients who say they just can't remember any more. I then ask them to pretend they are writing a short story (not a novel unless you have lots of time) and I ask what would they do next with the story. You also can ask them to be a screenwriter or a playwright. Ask them, if they could have their wish, would they write short stories, movie scripts, TV scripts or plays. Let them choose.

When we are negotiating and hit a firm resistance, I sometimes ask my patients/clients what they would do if I were the patient and they were the therapeutic facilitator. Since many patients/clients I see are healthcare professionals, this technique is especially effective. They can hardly resist the challenge, and they solve the problem.

I also use rapid-fire questions when I feel a resistance. I visualize that I am keeping the patient's defense off balance by doing so. The questions are usually about details, which also serve to strengthen the conscious-nonconscious communication line, as they concurrently prevent the reorganization of the resistance. I don't use this to overpower the resistance but only to get patients to answer before they think about it.

If you ask for an image and nothing comes after a reasonable time, ask the patient/client to imagine what an Inner Physician would be like if one did come, describe this imagined image, then imagine a dialogue with it. Soon they will be into the process. A further extension of this approach (which I seldom use) that can be very helpful in very resistant cases is to have the patient/client draw a picture of an Inner Physician if such a person did exist. You can go from there because you have the image started.

If an image won't talk, ask it why it won't talk. Ask how you can change conditions so that it might be willing to talk. Or perhaps it wishes to communicate in another way, such as telepathically or by providing mental pictures of answers and so on. Whatever the image wants to do is usually okay with me.

Another thing to remember: Ask your patients/clients to do all their talking aloud if they will. This seems to help overcome resistance as well as strengthen conscious/nonconscious communications. It is embarrassing at first but it is the quickest way to get past the negative conditioning most of us have been subjected to about daydreams, imaginings and talking to ourselves.

DIALOGUE STYLE AND CHOICE OF WORDS

Improper dialogue style and poor choice of words can impair the progress of therapeutic imagery and dialogue just as much as the improper use of the hands or a
wrong attitude. You must be ever alert and sensitive to the patient/client's response
to your style of speech, your tone of voice and your choice of words. The patient/
client response can be seen by facial and body expression; it can be heard in the
tone of voice and it can be felt with your hands.

When you are talking to a child character from the patient/client's
nonconscious, use simple words and phrases; be very literal. Identify with that
child, be a child with him or her unless it seems therapeutically beneficial to assume an authoritarian role. When the nonconscious character who presents is a
tough, streetwise person, be tough and streetwise with it; be like it. If you can't do
that, then admire the toughness and competency. The characters will be subject to
flattery, to admiration and probably will respond favorably if you ask for their help.
If the nonconscious character is a prim and proper person, respect that; be gentle,
very courteous and so on. The message is, "Do what you would need to do in daily
life to befriend and work with that kind of personality." Adapt your style to the
nonconscious character. Change your tone of voice, admire, push, be agreeable, be
a Martian if you need to be. Do whatever it takes to draw the character out and
gain its assistance. (Some of you may need to go to acting school to change your
persona as needed.) Remember, "When in Rome, do as the Romans do."

Your choice of words also can facilitate or obstruct the process of therapeutic
facilitation. Some words automatically carry optimistic, constructive connotations.
Other words carry pessimistic, defeatist, destructive, hypercritical baggage with
them. Choose your words to help you get the kind of effect you want. Usually, you
will need the optimistic constructive effect, but on some occasions you may desire
to magnify the destructive or negative aspect of the situation. In either case, be
aware that your choice of words will greatly influence the tone and progression of
the session.

There are literally thousands of examples whereby word choice sets the mood.
Often you, as the therapeutic facilitator, betray your mood by your choice of words.
As an example, when a nonconscious character says it is having a cup of tea, you
might ask if the tea is "nice and warm and steamy" which carries a pleasant connotation. Or you might ask if the tea is "hot" which opens the door for an unpleasant
burning association. When a patient sees clouds on the horizon you might ask if
they are "beautiful white billowy clouds." These words produce a nice feeling. Or
you might ask if they are "dark rain clouds." They might even be storm clouds and
feel threatening.

It is amazing to me how many dialoguers ask if they are storm clouds. This
suggestion most likely reflects what is on their personal horizon at that time. Why

not just ask the patient what kind of clouds they see? Let the patients tell you how they feel instead of you telling them how you feel. Actually, you don't need to categorize the clouds; you could just ask how the patient feels when he/she looks at the clouds. Don't ask how the clouds *make* them feel. We are trying to foster self-determination. You can help this cause by asking how the patient feels when he/she is looking at the clouds. You can work against self-determination by asking how the clouds make them feel.

Think about the connotations carried by some of the paired words that follow and see how they can be used or misused. You could be alert or anxious, open or undecided, self-assured or egotistical, trusting or gullible, laid-back or lazy, mild or meek, tenacious or stubborn—and so on until you exhaust the dictionary. Each of the first words in the preceding pairs carries a positive connotation and the second word in each pair carries some derogatory baggage. Each of the words in the pair has essentially the same meaning if we delete the connotation that it carries. So, please consider your words carefully and use them to help set the tone. You might even substitute positively connotated words for negatively connotated words used by the patient when you want to build confidence and self-esteem. For example, if patients/clients say they are "stubborn" you might say that it is the "tenacious" person who gets the job done. Or if they say they are "so gullible" you might comment that "trust" is wonderful. There should be more of it in this world.

I'm sure you get the idea. I suggest that you practice with words. Take a paragraph of dialogue from a play or novel. See how you can change the words to change the mood while preserving the story. Enjoy and apply what you discover to your dialogue techniques.

RELAXATION, DEEPENING AND STRENGTHENING

Initial induction of patient/client relaxation to the level in which productive thera-peutic imagery and dialogue can be carried out may be done by any number of methods.

The use of the CV-4 technique with relaxation intent in mind will often ac-complish the relaxation state without any words. This approach may be preferable for the patient who is wary of hypnosis, psychotherapy and the like. Once the state of relaxation is achieved (you can tell this with your hands), you can begin your imagery suggestions and dialogue. I used only the CV-4 for induction of relax-ation, therapeutic imagery and dialogue with 40 non-English-speaking Japanese in December 1988 during a SomatoEmotional Release course. It worked perfectly. If I had any doubts about the use of CV-4 with intention as a relaxation technique, they were dispelled in that class.

There are, of course, a wide range of relaxation techniques that involve verbal suggestion, eye fixation, breathing and other voluntary patient participation activi-ties. You can suggest that the body becomes relaxed and heavy. It is common to suggest that relaxation comes in through the feet. It feels very good. It ascends through the lower legs to the knees, through the thighs, to the hips and so on to the head and out the arms to the fingers. Go slowly. Mention many, many body parts and regions. Reinforce the pleasant, relaxed, heavy feeling frequently. Also frequently suggest that the tension is going out.

I have used eye fixation techniques often in the past but not as often in the last few years. In eye fixation, simply ask patients to intensely study a small object. Suggest that their eyes are getting tired, the focus goes in and out and finally that the lids get heavy and close. Go slowly. Repeat your statements and when the eyes close you can suggest that the body get very relaxed. You can suggest that all the body energy, which is in the form of tension, can be used by the eyes to study the object you have selected. I had a black spot on the ceiling of my treatment room to use as the object of eye fixation when I was using this technique. (This was B.C.S.T.—Before CranioSacral Therapy).

Many people use deep breathing to induce the consciousness state that fosters Therapeutic Imagery and Dialogue. I have seldom done this. I don't know why. I haven't used breathing much for relaxation induction or therapeutically. I know it works. I've had it done on me, but somehow it feels unnatural to me so I don't use it much yet. I may start tomorrow.

When I wish to deepen a state of relaxation or, more appropriately described, strengthen a nonconscious-conscious communication line, I usually have my pa-tients focus on the details of whatever image they see, feel, taste, smell or perceive in any way. The more details, the deeper the relaxation and the stronger the com-munication between conscious and nonconscious. For example, patients/clients will frequently get a visual image of a wise-looking old man when they ask for their Inner Physician to come forward. Let us say that the image is coming in and out of focus and that they do not get an answer when they ask the image if they may ask a few questions. These happenings suggest to me that the conscious-nonconscious communication line is open but the connection is tenuous.

To strengthen the conscious-nonconscious communication line, be sure that all requests and questions are spoken aloud by the patients/clients to the image(s). Encourage patients/clients to repeat the image's responses aloud. This mode of communication serves to deepen the relaxation state so that the imagery process is facilitated. As mentioned above, speaking aloud also overcomes initial resistance related to negative conditioning and embarrassment. You may need to offer a lot of encouragement to get some patients/clients to dialogue aloud with an image. If they cannot do it aloud, it tips you off to the fact that they need hands-on work for the mouth and throat. The fifth chakra also usually will need attention.

Once the patient/client is speaking aloud to the image, I like to direct the focus to details. This too may require a lot of encouragement from you. "You see the wise old man. Does he have a beard? You can see him; is there a beard? How long is the beard? Is it clipped and trimmed or is it uncut? What color is it? Can you see a mustache?" Ask about hair, shoes, sandals, height, weight, hands, ad infinitum. I usually save questions about the eyes until I'm sure the patient is comfortable with the image. Eyes can be scary if the patient has a fearsome image. Each detail you can get the patient/client to see strengthens the conscious-nonconscious communication lines.

After the details seem readily available and the dialogue is aloud without hesitation or embarrassment, I usually ask the patient/client to see if the image will speak directly to me through his/her voice. If the image says yes, then I ask the patient/client if it is okay that the image use his/her voice. Usually this is agreeable to the patient/client, but I feel better if the patient/client gives verbal assent out loud so the image can hear it.

Once you have obtained a situation of reasonably free flowing dialogue between the image, the patient and yourself, you will probably not need to further concern yourself with relaxation and deepening techniques. If the need does arise, I usually just go for more details or try to find out if a resistance is coming into the picture and requires attention.

DESENSITIZING TECHNIQUES

Most of the desensitizing techniques have been introduced previously in one place or another in this section of the book. I believe they should be brought together in one place. This is the place. Please forgive the repetition.

Essentially, desensitization refers to the process of becoming better and better acquainted with a fearsome and powerful situation. We use it in many aspects of practice. Recently, a patient I worked with off and on for more three years arrived in a state of near panic. Two days earlier she had been hit with a sudden onset of diarrhea followed by nausea and a little vomiting. Then her world began to spin incredibly. It was a true vertigo (the world spinning around you) that she described. Every time she changed her head position the world took off spinning. The nausea continued but the diarrhea never returned.

My tentative diagnosis was Meniere's disease, an inflammation of the semicircular canals in the petrous parts of the temporal bones. The endolymph thickens a bit, the cilia over-respond and the sensation of vertigo (the world spinning around you) is overwhelming. Whenever the victim moves his/her head the endolymph are stirred and stimulate the cilia, but they dysfunction and the victim feels dizzy.

I asked the patient to lie down on the table. She said she could not. She said that she had slept in a chair since this began. She was afraid to lie down because every time she tried, she became very "spinny" and sick to her stomach.

I used the desensitizing principle to get her to lie down. I had her sit with her feet on the table and my hands on her head. Then I had her lean back a few degrees—which changed her head's orientation to gravity—until she began to get a little dizzy. We waited until the dizziness cleared. I kept my hands on her head. When her equilibrium calmed down, as I supported her with my hands, I had her recline a little further until she wanted to stop again because of the return of the dizziness. We waited until her sense of equilibrium normalized. Then we went a little further toward the supine position until, again, she had to stop. Five or six repetitions of the stop-wait-go process brought us to the supine position where I could effectively work on her cranium. I taught her how to do her own gentle ear pull because the temporal bones are usually the chief offender in vertigo and Meniere's disease as far as the symptoms are concerned.

This was a process of desensitizing. Each time we moved her head in relation to the gravitational orientation of the earth, we went slowly and gently and the equilibrium system could handle just a little more. It became more and more accommodative of the movement. We went only as far as she would allow, then we stopped and waited until the endolymph and the cilia adjusted. Had we gone too far or moved quickly and forcibly, the ensuing panic both psychoemotionally and physiologically would have put us right back at square one. We would have had to overcome the resistance resultant to the bad experience before we could move on toward square two again.

I explained what was happening physiologically as I worked with her, and by the end of the session she went from a supine to a sitting position without assistance. She felt some vertigo. She waited for the adjustment of her equilibrium to occur without panic or fear. She then stood, went over to the chair, sat and waited for the vertigo to disappear. She bent forward and put on her shoes while she had some very mild "spinny" feelings. She chose not to wait for it to clear because she knew it would come back for a short time after she sat straight up. It did and she waited a moment. She then stood, smiled, said "thank you" and was on her way.

She was desensitized. She had became familiar with the physiological dysfunction. She accepted it. She knew what it would do and when. She could now deal with her symptoms without the incapacitating panic and fear that had taken charge of her.

Another good example of desensitization is the toe in the cold water first, then the foot, then both feet. Next, we go in up to the knees and the thighs. There is usually a longer wait before we get the pelvis and genitalia into cold water. Many of us then will dive into the water once the pelvis has accommodated. Some will go on inch by inch until they are swimming. This is desensitization. Most of us have done it. Some people do not desensitize and don't go into the water all the way. There is also a macho group that will dive into anything. (I suppose this is rapid desensitization but you do hear a lot of yelling and screaming when it is done suddenly.)

Desensitizing the patient/client for therapeutic imaging and dialogue is essentially the same in principle. We also desensitize when we're restoring joint motion. We gradually increase passive range of motion with many repetitions and to tolerance, then we may add active range of motion with lots of encouragement and assurance.

When we have a patient/client who is nonconsciously confronting a very powerful and fearsome experience, we have to try to take the power away from the experience. We try to desensitize by familiarizing the patient/client with an experience. When it happened, it was horrible. It was immediately locked away by the nonconscious protector in a strongbox. The protector keeps it there because it is too horrible to look at, but there is a rental fee for the strongbox and there is a salary for the nonconscious protector's services to guard it each month. The cost of fees and salaries might translate to nightmares every night, headaches every day, fear of strangers, acrophobia, chronic anger, mortal fear, pain anywhere in the body or anything else that you might dream of. There seems to be no limit except that which is self- imposed by the nonconscious.

How do you go about pulling the teeth out of such an experience? You must help the patient/client put it in a different perspective so that it is less fearsome. To do this, you usually must examine the experience in detail. Let's take an example that is one of the most fearsome and emotionally charged that I have ever encountered.

This woman, about 50 years of age, presented with unrelenting headaches. They were incapacitating for days at a time. The headaches had begun when she was in her late teens. They were then controllable with pain medications. When she was about 30 years of age, the medication didn't work any more. She went into psychotherapy and had been in it for about 20 years when she came to us for evaluation.

She went into S.E.R. on the first visit and it seemed that the headaches were a symptom under the control of a nonconscious part of her that was insisting on attention. The message was that she was sane, she must face the truth, she must trust her memories and not the denials of her parents. Memories of what? We couldn't even approach the material directly.

I developed a good speaking rapport and friendship with her headaches. The headaches then became the responsibility of an angel named Sam. Sam and I became quite close. We could dialogue without the patient/client being consciously aware of our conversation, and so I finally convinced Sam to share with me what it was that was locked away in the patient's strongbox and was so well protected.

Sam told me that childhood sexual abuse began at less than a year of age and continued until the age of nine. The abuse included the mother, the father and a string of deranged and perverted "nannies." There was excessive use of enema tubes, masturbation of the child by the parents, and then, when old enough, masturbation and fellatio of the father by the child with the mother instructing. The nannies did not seem to be invited into most of these sessions, but usually did preparatory work with the enema equipment that was supposed to erotically stimulate the child.

Sam said that the patient could probably handle knowledge of this material although, to date, she had denied that it had happened. The one incident that Sam felt was important to accept as fact was as follows: The patient was four years old. The mother and father were trying to achieve an insertion of the father's erect penis into the four-year-old vagina of the patient. It was not going well because the vagina was too small. After a few unsuccessful attempts at insertion, the mother took a scissors and cut the tissues of her daughter's vagina so the orifice was enlarged enough to accommodate at least a portion of the father's penis. Intercourse was then carried to climax by the father. It was at this time that the mother got a little worried that a doctor might get suspicious. The story was invented that she fell on a pipe that protruded from the ground as part of an old swing set in the backyard. Blood was smeared on the pipe in case there was an investigation.

It was then that the brainwashing of the patient began by the mother and the father. Although the sexual abuse continued for another four or five years, the parents felt secure in their secret because they had convinced their daughter that none of it was real, it was all her fantasy. They told her she was insane and that if she told anyone of her insane fantasies they would have to put her in an asylum. But as long as she didn't tell anyone, they would keep the secret of her insanity and she could live at home. Sam gave her headaches so that she would get attention and hopefully discover that she was sane, that these memories were real and that her parents were sick, not she.

Well, how do you begin desensitizing something like this? First, I had to let go of my repulsion. Then I began by seeing if there were other parts of her nonconsciousness that I could connect with. It turned out that there were several who were eager to talk. There was, of course, the little girl who tearfully described the events that had been previously described for me by Sam. The little girl gave me more detail. I realized that this was part of the desensitization process although the patient was not consciously aware yet of our discussions. Sam had accomplished the first step toward desensitization. Then, the little girl went further with more detail.

I went through the experiences with the little girl on several occasions, each time in more detail than the time before and with less fear. I helped the little girl to realize that it was okay to come out of hiding, that her parents were mentally ill, that she would not go to the asylum for telling what had happened. And, I put her under the loving care of Sam the angel.

Next, I went to the protector and began trying to convince him that, in small doses, perhaps the adult patient could handle the truth about her childhood. The protector was definitely the protector; he was very cautious. He held the key to the strongbox where the horrible memories were locked away. He softened a little but would not yet let any of these experiences come to conscious awareness. I worked with the protector some at each session. I made sure that he was aware of the patient's progress toward truth.

Next, I met "Duke." He was the angry, aggressive one. He was, by description, physically reminiscent to me of The Fonz (Henry Winkler) on the television show *Happy Days*. Duke was tough and wanted to avenge the abuse but he was not tough enough to go after mother or father. He did kick the nannies on occasion. Once, when a nanny was coming with the enema bag, Duke had the eight-year-old girl hide a scissors under the mattress. As Nanny pinned our eight-year-old patient's face down on the bed and prepared for anal insertion of the tube, Duke reached around the mattress, grabbed the scissors and stabbed Nanny in the thigh. The woman ran out of the room screaming and resigned her position that night. The incident was denied by the mother and father. They said it was a dream. (Is it any wonder this patient was holding on to her sanity by a headache that was under the control of an angel named Sam?)

There were, after this, several little girls of different ages who came forward, each with her own story of different abuse scenarios. It really tested my ability to be non-judgmental and to believe in the Significance Detector that told me that all this material was significant and, I believe, real.

After several sessions in which the patient began to get partial conscious awareness of some material as the protector let it out of his strongbox, I asked the patient to write a story about a little girl who was growing up in a home similar to her own. This was further desensitization. She wove bits and pieces of her life into her story. Then we converted her story to a screenplay and imagined that we were watching the movie together. There were more details of her childhood as the movie progressed. Then, I asked if she could play the lead in her movie. She finally agreed, and as she played the part she was further desensitized.

Finally, all at once, about the fourth time she played the part, she looked me right in the eye and said, "That movie is about me and that little girl is me and that is what happened to me." She then said that she wasn't crazy and she finally knew it. Her headaches greatly improved. This was a tough bit of reality to swallow. When she allowed self-doubt to creep in, her headache came back. When she felt sure it had all happened and trusted her sanity, the headache went away. She knew what her headache was about and what her life was about. All this progress occurred over a period of four months and 28 sessions.

Her father was dead by this time. Her mother was alive and remarried. She decided to visit her mother. While with her mother, her reality contact softened and her headaches came back with a vengeance. She couldn't believe her mother could have done all this horrible stuff to her. As the self-doubt increased, the headaches increased. She came back again with moderate headaches that became the standard when she is away from her mother.

The problem is not totally resolved. She still has times when she can't believe that this really happened to her. We have more work to do. Perhaps she needs time to digest her insights and then will be able to work with them herself. But I believe she will require a great deal of help. In any case, she has had a look at her life and can see her reflection in her mirror.

This is the most difficult case I ever tried to desensitize. Most are much easier. But it has to be helpful for you to know that we all have problem patients. The desensitizing techniques illustrated in this patient interaction just about run the gamut of techniques I use:

1. Nonconscious characters can recount experiences without the patient/client's conscious awareness hearing the dialogue. This desensitizes to some extent.

2. Have the patient/client write a story about someone who is like he or she was when the experience occurred. They need not know about the experience yet.

3. Have patients/clients distance themselves and watch the experience from the ceiling. Repeat it, having them stay in the body as a participant over and over as long as possible, then jump out of their bodies when they need to. Repeat the experience, having them stay in as a participant over and over as long as possible, until patients/clients finally participate in their bodies all the way through the experience. Do it a few more times until you see signs of boredom. Then try to get them to see some humor related to the session and laugh with you about it.

4.   If they can't get out of their bodies when it gets tough during the experience, go back to the beginning of the experience. Let them watch it on a movie or television screen. Big is more potent and color is more potent, so you may have to start on a small black and white television screen. Then, when they can do the whole experience on a small black and white TV, bring in color and do it again. When this is done, bring in larger screens all the way up to the wraparound movie screen in vivid color.

5.   You may find it beneficial to ask patients to be actors in the television show or movie as they view it. And remember, you can ask them to write the script.

6.   Prioritizing, a technique not mentioned or used in the preceding case, is simply a question of revaluing the injured body. Many abuse patients become obsessed with the desecration of their body. I try to get them to understand that their body can still serve them even though it has been defiled—just as I can still take my car to work even with a dented fender. Or, I can cry over the fender and not go to work. If you want to see people who overvalue their bodies, go to Muscle Beach or to a Narcissus contest. In any case, I try to get patients to see that their bodies can still serve them even though they have been raped, sodomized or had an extremity amputated.

7.   Use your imagination. Improvise. You understand the principle of desensitization; use it. Ultimately, you want patients to relive the experience in detail from beginning to end, over and over again until it becomes commonplace for them.

8.   Always go for humor near the end. If patients can laugh at any part of the experience, they are laughing at themselves. If they can laugh at themselves, they won't take themselves and life quite so seriously. This is definitely desensitizing and therapeutic.

ACCEPTANCE AND FORGIVENESS

Once suppressed materials, experiences, memories, emotions and the like come into conscious awareness, there is often the issue of what to do about the wrong that someone may have done to the patient. It could be a drunk driver who killed a loved one or who maimed or injured the patient or a loved one. It could be a swindler, a rapist, a murderer. It could be an abusive parent or sibling. It could be God for dealing the patient a bad hand in this lifetime.

In alternative and New Age work, it is common to work toward forgiveness of a fellow human being who has somehow hurt, damaged or offended one. It is also reasonably common to work toward acceptance of the trials and tribulations attributed to God. I remember how angry I was with God when he allowed my father to die shortly after my thirteenth birthday. I couldn't imagine how a "loving God" could do that. Now I accept that it happened and can find a rational reason. Acceptance is defined as the state of accepting or being accepted. Among other definitions offered in *Webster's Unabridged Dictionary:* To accept is to take or receive what is offered with a consenting mind; to understand. "Forgiveness," is defined in the same dictionary as the state of forgiving or a pardon. To forgive is to give up resentment or the desire to punish, to stop being angry with. Both words and the acts or states of mind that they represent are often misunderstood.

Many people think of acceptance as hopeless resignation. This is not so. Acceptance means that you take what comes and see what you can do about it without exercising anger or feeling vengeful. If you believe in reincarnation, you will probably be able to accept what comes—be it pleasant or unpleasant—as part of a greater plan. Thus, you may consider every adverse situation, every accident, disease and loss is a lesson. These adversities are challenges to be used to stimulate new growth and evolution. Be careful that your patients/clients do not confuse acceptance with resignation and hopelessness.

True forgiveness is accepting, non-judgmental, penetrates all levels and parts of the nonconscious and is filled with love. It is not a "well, I guess so" act with reservations attached. Forgiveness is a word we often use incorrectly. I hear, "I forgive him," used repeatedly in a condescending way. To some people, the ability to forgive implies that the forgiver possesses superior power over the forgivee. In this setting, forgiveness contributes to a hierarchy of "good" and "bad." Forgivers in these circumstances pardon the one who they feel has hurt them, much as a governor pardons a criminal. The governor holds life and death or at least imprisonment power over the offender.

I try to be very careful not to contribute to this somewhat trite and hierarchical situation. Therefore, I do not use the word "forgiveness" very often. I use it only when I feel sure it is used correctly, from one human peer to another or from one spiritual being to another. I believe that all earthbound humans have flaws and weaknesses, otherwise we wouldn't be here. We also have strengths and talents. When you have been wronged by another, you have encountered one of his/her flaws or weaknesses.

This may have been scripted before either of you was born or it may have happened that you were just there when the weakness or flaw ventilated. This ventilation could result in an act of violence, robbery or deception or the like. Remember that you too have weaknesses and flaws, and but for the grace of God the situation could be reversed. You could be the hurter and the other person could be the hurtee. What I mean by this is that we are all imperfect beings. We should accept each other's imperfections. We should not condescend to someone who has demonstrated an imperfection and perhaps injured us. We should recognize that we too are imperfect. We may have strengths and weaknesses in different areas so that we don't physically assault anyone, but we could be doing or have done just as much emotional damage to a loved one when we were constantly on their case about something.

Forgiveness is wonderful but don't let the self-righteous patient use it to continue or create a "holier than thou" attitude. This happens a lot and it simply creates further problems. Forgiveness is an acceptance that both the parties involved are imperfect and it could have been the other way around. Frequently, the part that people discover later is that it was the other way around at another time.

Do not take sides and support a self-righteous attitude in the patient. This is counterproductive. The most dramatic example I have encountered that illustrates the inhibition of therapeutic progress by the therapist agreeing with the self-righteous patient is well worth reciting to you now.

The patient was a 40-year-old woman who began working with me to alleviate a temporomandibular joint syndrome. She was in mouth splints and had been in braces. SomatoEmotional Release began during the first session and it became clear that she had been sexually involved with her father as a child. The act that was repeatedly committed was fellatio and it came right up during the first SomatoEmotional Release. She said that it was true and that she had been in psychotherapy and counseling off and on for many years to get past the damage her father had done. She felt very angry, self-righteous and defiled. Her therapists through the years had supported the wrongness of her father's deeds and helped keep her in the role of victim.

After the first SomatoEmotional Release, I instinctively knew there was more to the sexual relationship with her father than she had uncovered during her years of therapy because the issue was at the top of her nonconscious agenda. At subsequent sessions we used Therapeutic Imagery and Dialogue with SomatoEmotional Release. We went through sexual experiences with her father and with an adult neighbor detail by detail. The experiences began when she was just a few months old. Her father used to fondle her genitalia as he masturbated himself. At age three, the fellatio began with her father and at age eight she performed fellatio on an adult male neighbor through the fence between their adjoining yards. She charged the neighbor man 25 cents for this service.

What we got in touch with that the other therapists had missed was that she enjoyed the sex with her father. She re-experienced the pleasant sensations and emotions during our sessions. She was astonished at the enjoyment which later included a sense of power over her father during the act of fellatio. She tried to gain power over the adult male neighbor in the same way. As an infant, when her father sexually fondled her, it was pleasurable. She felt no shame, guilt or sense of being abused. Her father loved her and what he did felt good. As time went on, he introduced her to his penis that he had been fondling himself during their time together. She began to fondle his penis as he instructed her to do. She was fascinated by how it changed size and squirted out white sticky stuff if she did it right. Ultimately, her father let her know how good it tasted and taught her to perform fellatio. This became almost a daily ritual.

Mother worked the afternoon shift at a hospital as a nurse's aide. Father worked days, so they were conveniently alone together most evenings. As she got a little older, she began to realize the she had power over her authoritarian father during the time of fellatio. She felt the power and enjoyed it.

She loved it so much that she tried to extend her power to the neighbor man, and he rewarded her with a quarter. At age eight, her parent's marriage dissolved and her father left home. That was the end of fellatio for a few years, but she began again as a young teenager. She was searching for control and rewards from the boys.

Her therapists had automatically placed her in the victim role. They told her how badly she had been treated by her father and that he was a scoundrel. By making the father the abuser and her the victim, they did not allow room for her to remember the pleasure and sense of power that she felt. This therapeutic approach fostered powerful guilt because her nonconscious knew of her pleasure. The guilt then suppressed the pleasant memories and kept her in an emotionally destructive mode. She had tried to forgive her father but couldn't really find a reason why she must do so because he had given her a lot of pleasure and love.

If her previous therapists had not taken sides, this patient might have realized much sooner that both she and her father were imperfect. She could have been helped to accept pleasures that an infant and young girl did not consider as wrong and her enjoyment of her sexual experiences and her use of fellatio to exercise power and control. Her father had taught her it was good behavior right from the beginning. Then, society told her that if she did those things she was bad. A lot of powerful internal conflict developed. She then tried to blame her father for her evil deeds and this was later supported by her therapists. How could she admit that what was so bad actually felt so good and gave her power? She had to pull it out and look at it. She had to feel guilt and rationalize her behavior. She had to accept herself and her father as they were then and as they are now. Don't take sides.

Her temporomandibular joint syndrome is gone now. Yes, it did relate to the fellatio. As she discovered it was wrong in the eyes of society and in the eyes of her therapists, she was less and less able to open her mouth widely. The constant hypertonicity of the jaw muscles created some inflammation of the joints. The guilt gone, the jaws relaxed and she healed wonderfully well.

So, it is important to be cautious about misusing acceptance and forgiveness—and about taking sides.

RESOLUTION AND APPLICATION IN EVERYDAY LIFE

Once you go through all this catharsis and re-experiencing and gaining of insight with patients, what do you do with it? How does it change their lives?

First, I believe that the opening of communication lines between the patient/client's conscious awareness and the various regions of the nonconscious is the most important thing that can happen. Develop a program to help keep them open. Have the patient/client set up a time every day when the various characters who have come forward from the nonconsciousness will meet with the patient's conscious awareness. This should be a pleasant meeting. It is very effective right upon awakening before getting out of bed. Set up a system of signals to be given if the patient begins to neglect the meetings. I frequently suggest the return of a familiar symptom that the patient consciously recognizes is controlled by the nonconscious. This could be an abdominal cramp, an epigastric pain, a jab of sciatic pain or anything that is mutually agreeable to the nonconscious and the conscious. This works really well, with about the same potency as a posthypnotic suggestion.

Acceptance of what happened is important. Now that it is over, let's extract the lessons from the experience and move forward. Let's get on with life and growth and healing. There is no place for self-pity, remorse, anger, resentment nor a need for vengeance. Keep working with your patients/clients until they either let it all go or refuse to do so. If they refuse, be sure that you have tried to help them see the cost of the destructive feelings they harbor.

Self-realization will usually change a patient/client's life. I used to think that I had to help them change, but when healing is done, let it be done. Watch what happens. Trust it. Don't go back and worry or fret. Don't try to redo it. You have therapeutically facilitated the enhancement of self-awareness and knowledge. The enhanced self-awareness makes your patients/clients better able to deal with what will come up tomorrow. They are more independent. They don't need you. How does that feel to you? It should feel good.

Chapter VI
Personal Growth
Experiences

Many people follow great teachers who facilitate their education and growth. I have been given examples and cast into situations. My teachers are present but they seem less tangible than most. The most important lesson they seem to offer is to be open and observe.

John E. Upledger, D.O., O.M.M

ACUPUNCTURE: A REAL EYE OPENER

In 1967 we opened two free clinics in Pinellas County, Florida. One was in St. Petersburg and the other one in Clearwater. We treated a variety of needy people including wonderful poor people, derelicts, young people in need of birth control and sex counseling and a whole crop of drug abusers and addicts. We were, of course, always looking for ways to cut costs.

Butch, who was one of our clinic directors, had gone to San Francisco for a seminar for free clinic directors. He returned with a small paperbound book that was a manual for pain control. It was originally written for North Korean barefoot doctors as a field manual. It was translated to English before Nixon went to China. So acupuncture was not yet a popular topic of conversation in the U.S. Butch showed me this little manual, and I shrugged it off. Butch hit me in the ego/pride by saying, "John, you're supposed to be open-minded. Why won't you try this? If it works we could save a lot on medicine in the clinics."

So I read the booklet. It was about 40 pages with several illustrations, and in the last chapter were nine points to needle that would relieve pain anywhere in the body. These needles, when inserted, were supposed to be comparable in analgesic potency to a quarter grain of morphine. The benefit was that the needles would not interfere with mental action as did the morphine. These needles had been used to ease the pain of wounded soldiers so that they could be transported to medical facilities and still have their wits about them.

I was pretty skeptical but Butch kept after me until finally I agreed to try it on three very difficult pain patients. One patient was a young man with acute rheumatoid arthritis who was in a lot of pain. The second patient was a man in his sixties with bone cancer metastatic to the lumbar spine from the prostate gland who was also in constant and severe pain. The third patient was an alcoholic woman in her late fifties with chronic pain in the area of the liver and biliary duct system. She also had bile in her urine almost constantly. I had dried her out in the hospital some months prior. She also had gallstones. So we surgically removed her gallbladder and the stones. We had also explored her bile and hepatic duct systems but could find no more stones or other problems. I felt that the bile in the urine was due to residual liver disease from long years of alcohol abuse, but we had no answer for her continuous acute pain.

I thought these three patients would be an effective challenge to the nine magic needle placements described in the little booklet. If the pain was relieved, acupuncture would have my attention. If it was not relieved, Butch agreed to get off my back.

I used 25-gauge disposable hypodermic needles. With the book in one hand and a needle in the other, I put nine needles in each of these three patients. Each needle went in about half an inch. I'm sure I inspired a lot of confidence as I read the book, mumbled under my breath and jabbed with a needle. The plan was to leave the needles in place for about 30 minutes. I know that you are just dying to know where the needles were placed. The points were:

Large intestine 4 – bilateral
Stomach 36 – bilateral
Gallbladder 36 – bilateral
Pericardium 4 – bilateral
Governing vessel 16.

Within 10 minutes the rheumatoid arthritis patient said his pain was all gone. He remained in pain remission for two days, then the pain returned. He would not come in for another treatment. (My suspicion was that being pain-free scared the hell out of him—as much as did my obvious amateur status as an acupuncturist.)

The cancer patient got about 75 percent relief of pain within 30 minutes. I showed his wife, a Licensed Practical Nurse, where and how to insert the needles. I marked the points with a skin pencil. She needled him twice a day as he needed it, always using the same points and the 25-gauge disposable needles. He lived about two months. He needed no narcotics. He did very well with the needles as his pain control method until he died.

The third patient was most remarkable. She was pain free by the time I got the last needle in place. She remained pain free for 24 hours. Even more remarkable, the color of her urine changed from a bile-stained greenish-yellow to a normal color for about two days. She came in for follow-up treatments about three times a week.

After some experimentation I finally found that I could insert one needle just below the inferior costal margin about five inches to the right of the anterior midline of the body (I didn't know anything about meridians or Chinese inches at that time) and achieve pain relief for a few hours. This was easier than using all of the nine needles. I left this one needle in place with antibiotic cream on the puncture site and a bandage over it for three days. The urine remained clear of bile while the needle was in place, but the bile returned about eight or nine hours after I took the needle out. I needed to find something besides a needle to stimulate this area. The needle did the job systemically but it was too irritating. I put a rather heavy gauge silk suture through this point and tied a little chain onto it—the type found on old- fashioned drain plugs. I put antibiotic cream over the suture, covered it with a large band-aid and let the chain hang down. I told her whenever she had the pain to pull the chain intermittently until the pain stopped. I was just guessing. I asked her to change the bandage every day, clean the area with peroxide and apply fresh antibiotic cream.

After about two weeks of chain pulling, the time between pulls became longer and longer. Finally, the pain didn't return and the urine stayed clear. The patient was totally recovered. Never able to pay her bill, she made drapes for the office. She taught me a lot about open-mindedness, not being afraid to try what seems to make sense and the fact that in modern medicine we are really only scratching the surface. We stayed in touch with each other for at least five years after her remarkable recovery. Her liver and bile duct system problems did not surface again clinically during all of that time. To my knowledge, she never used ethanol again. She was certainly a great teacher.

ACUPUNCTURE OPENS MY MIND AND MY EYES FURTHER

I had a few more really eye-opening and mind-expanding experiences with acupuncture in the late sixties. After that first experience with the pain alleviation which led to my observation that a silk suture in the right place might restore a liver to normal function, I was moved to do some study of the acupuncture system. I found an Oriental bookstore catalogue through the San Francisco-based Free Clinic Association. A British internist, Felix Mann, had authored four books on the subject. I felt that any British internal medicine specialist who could write four books on the subject must be pretty good, so I sent for and received Dr. Mann's four books.

I didn't have them more than a week when a patient came in with acute herpes zoster (shingles). The lesions where full blown all around the course of the seventh intercostal nerve on the right side. The patient was a 25-year-old woman who was almost hysterical from the pain (probably in some part due to the fact that she was prone to hysteria). She came to see me after her family doctor had injected cortisone and it hadn't helped. A friend told her that I was good with difficult problems. I looked at the rash and knew that it hurt a lot. I tried to palpate the rib angles and vertebrae in the mid-thoracic area and she almost fainted.

Then it came. Eureka!!!! Let's try acupuncture.

I had read Dr. Mann's books once. There was no index, so I started looking through the contents of *Acupuncture: Treatment of Many Diseases*. I found what I was looking for about two-thirds of the way through the totally disorganized table of contents. "Intercostal Neuralgia" (pages 121 and 122) "... use liver 4, 13 and 14 bilateral, bladder 17 and 18 bilateral and pericardium 6 bilateral points for left-sided pain. Use liver 14 (right side only), bladder 18 bilateral, conception vessel 12 and 17, pericardium 6 (right side only), stomach 40 (left side only), gallbladder 40 (left side only) and spleen 17 (right side only) points for right-sided pain." There was no explanation about how the treatment points had been selected.

I extended Dr. Mann the courtesy of trust and used the points for the right-sided pain. I inserted the 25-gauge disposable hypodermic needles. Some bled and some didn't. Within minutes her pain subsided significantly. The redness of the rash blanched out as I watched it. She became totally pain free as I sat on my stool and watched. Her hysteria subsided. I structurally corrected the mid-thoracic vertebrae and mobilized the ribs using thrust technique.

I treated her five more times using the same acupuncture points and direct thrust manipulative technique. That was the end of the herpes zoster. My treatment schedule was based on how she felt. She called me every day to report how things were going. She was eternally grateful.

In short order I was bombarded with more than 30 cases of herpes zoster within the next few months. It worked so well that I was literally propelled into a very busy acupuncture practice in a few short weeks.

There are three more acupuncture experiences that I must relate because they were so mind expanding. First is the case of a 48-year-old nurse who suffered a brain tumor. The tumor had been removed by the neurosurgeon at our hospital, but she developed acute facial pain after the surgery. The surgeon called to ask if I would try acupuncture on her. I agreed with the caveat that it would be exploratory.

Out came the—by now famous and trusted—manual of Felix Mann, M.D. I looked up facial pain and added a few of my own ideas about opening exit points to release the pain from the meridia that passed through the painful areas. (By then I had some smaller 27-gauge disposable needles to use.) The Bladder 1 is placed at about the same spot where the nose piece for eyeglasses rests. I put in all of the other needles and told her I'd be back in 10 minutes to see how she was doing. I had a busy office and it was my practice to treat several patients at the same time.

When I came back to remove the needles, the one in Bladder 1 on the painful right side had been drawn into the tissue up to its nub and its point was aimed directly at the eyeball. Originally, I had just barely penetrated the deep side of the skin with this needle and the point was aimed at the nose when I left. (Incidentally, the Bladder 1 needle on the nonpainful left side was still as I had placed it.) I asked if she had tampered with the needles. She denied having done so and I really had no reason to disbelieve her. (After all, who would want to put a needle into her eyeball?) I gently tried to retract the needle from its position and direction of point. It would not budge. I tapped, I twirled, I wiggled the needle. Nothing helped. I removed the other needles. Bladder 1 on the right showed no sign of loosening. I decided I would have to use brute force. It was like pulling a really tough weed. Finally it came out.

There was tissue attached to the last half centimeter of the needle. This attached tissue I had to deliver through a hole in the skin that was much too small. It was only the needle shaft that had gone in through the hole. With the tissue attached, the needle diameter was now at least four times that of the original penetrating shaft.

I sent the needle to the pathology department at the hospital. The pathologist called me to ask what I was doing at my office. He reported that the needle had had a rather large quantity of fibrous connective and muscle tissue fused to it. He said it appeared to have been fused to the metal by either heat or electricity. He used the analogy of meat being fused to a skewer after it has been cooked over an open pit. He had not seen anything like this before he said. I told him I hadn't either. There was no heat or electricity used in this treatment. In fact, I doubt that I had even touched the metal needle shaft because I always held only the plastic nub of the disposable needle in order to make the insertion.

This experience certainly made a statement about energy within the body—

and about not being dependent upon external sources. I've not seen this happen since this first experience, but I certainly cannot dismiss this observation simply because I have not seen it twice. The patient's facial pain was due to an infection in the maxillary sinus. After it was opened and drained, she responded well to acupuncture treatment.

The next astonishment that I experienced was a case of secondary heart failure that was not responding to traditional medical care. Harold was a big, robust, happy man in his late sixties. I had been his family doctor for a couple of years. Suddenly, for no reason I could discover, he began to suffer episodes of acute shortness of breath, cardiac arrhythmia, fluid retention and the whole syndrome that we call cardiac asthma. He was hospitalized four times in three months via the emergency room. During his fourth hospitalization, I asked for help from cardiology because I was getting nowhere. At the end of this hospitalization Harold went home with digitalis to control his heart ventricles, quinidine to control the atria of his heart, six lasix a day to get rid of his excess body fluid, prednisone to help keep his lungs clear, an inhaler to use when he got short of breath and an oxygen tank in his living room, just in case.

He came to the office about three days after being discharged from the hospital. He told me that if this was how he had to live, he would rather die. I didn't much blame him although I did not want him to die—and not only because it was a terrible way to live: He was a fun guy and I really liked him, and also we hadn't solved his problem as yet and curiosity is a great motivator. He asked about "this here acupuncture" that he heard I was fooling around with. I told him that I had no idea how to treat him with acupuncture. He said he trusted me and that he was sure I could figure out what to do. How could I refuse?

I had been fooling around with Chinese pulse diagnosis as described by Felix Mann. I had accepted that acupuncture needling worked, but diagnosis by pulse seemed preposterous to me. Nonetheless, Dr. Mann said it was reliable, so I examined Harold's pulses. Oddly enough, his heart and lung pulses seemed full and vital. I couldn't find his kidney pulse. My surprise was probably on my face. Harold encouraged me to "go for it." I did.

I put needles in kidney tonification, kidney associated, kidney source, kidney alarm and any other kidney stimulation points I could discover on Dr. Mann's chart. I did nothing else except tell Harold to come back in 24 hours and bring all of his urine with him in a clean gallon milk jug.

The next day at 2 p.m., Harold came in cussing and raising hell in a good humored way I hadn't seen him display in four or five months. He announced to those in the waiting room that he hadn't slept all night because he was up "pissin." Harold had almost two gallons of urine that he had produced during the night; he had lost 16 pounds overnight according to our scales. He felt great.

Harold remained in my practice until I left for Michigan in 1975. He never had another problem with his heart, lungs or kidneys. He even had uneventful lumbar disc surgery in 1973. His heart did fine.

This was certainly another mind expanding experience for me. I have trusted the pulses and my ability to use them ever since. In his previous hospital admissions, Harold showed no signs of kidney problems. It all seemed to be heart and lungs. The pulses contradicted our Western diagnosis. I never had to treat Harold's kidneys by acupuncture or any other method again. Once was enough. His kidney pulses were palpable the next day. I weaned him from his medicine over about a week's time and we turned in his oxygen tank.

I sure didn't know what to make of this. How could the position and pressure of a finger on the radial artery tell if a guy like Harold had heart, lung or kidney problems as his primary problem? You tell me. We just weren't equipped to understand this in our society. So much to learn. Thank you, Harold.

The next acupuncture experience that further expanded my mind and increased my humility was presented by Linda. Linda was a very attractive, young, single woman in her mid-twenties. She was an upward bound, successful professional in the legislative branch of state government. Linda presented with a very acute case of genital herpes (before it was a popular "in" disease). The labia of the vagina were very red and terribly swollen. She could not bear to have anything touch this area of her body, including underwear. Her acute pain and distress prompted me to try steroid and local anesthetic injections into the lower sacral regions. I was trying to treat the triggers to the area. I did relevant osteopathic manipulation and provided her with a topical anesthetic spray which I hoped would ease the pain and perhaps interrupt the segmental facilitation.

She was back in two days. She was no better and perhaps a little worse, if that were possible. I really didn't know what to do. Then it struck me, "Let's try acupuncture." Again, I looked through Dr. Mann's table of contents in *Acupuncture: Treatment of Many Diseases* but could find nothing relevant. Then I remembered that in one of his other books Dr. Mann stated that the Chinese view pain as "fire." So, I decided that I needed to let the fire out of the kidney and bladder meridians that controlled and/or passed through the painful areas. (These would be the kidney and bladder meridians.)

I used the fire points to loosen or mobilize the pain on the meridians. I used the exit points to let the fire pain out of the meridian once it was mobilized. And I used the source points because my understanding was that they would act homeostatically, letting chi (energy) in or out depending on what was appropriate. I felt that letting all of that fire/pain energy out might have drained the meridian but I wasn't sure, so I used the source point. I figured that I would let the acupuncture point decide what was appropriate because I certainly did not know what I was doing. Once again, I used the disposable hypodermic needles bilaterally in the fire, exit and source points of both the kidney and bladder meridians.

Within minutes of the needle insertion, Linda's pain began to subside. I had her positioned on the gynecology table with her feet and legs in stirrups so that I could observe the vaginal labia. The labial swelling began to reduce. I could touch the labia without Linda screaming in agony. Within 30 minutes the pain and swelling were at least 80 percent gone.

I treated Linda three more times on consecutive days. When we finished the third follow-up treatment, there were no more subjective symptoms although I could still see a little minor swelling of the labia majora. I did pelvic and Pap smears for her every six months for about two years after this episode. There was no recurrence of the herpes during that time.

What next? Now you can let pain out of the body like turning on a faucet.

YOUR WHOLE BODY IS ON YOUR EAR?

I had accepted and used body acupuncture successfully. I had been astonished to see the diagnostic reliability of pulse diagnosis. Now I was presented with the ridiculous idea that your whole body is represented on your ear. I had just read a book entitled *Auriculotherapy* by French physician Paul F. M. Nogier, M.D. He described the homunculus on the ear. He explained that the ear cartilage represented the bones of the spine; the soft tissue distalward to the ear cartilage was the paravertebral muscle and that the outer edge of the ear represented the spinal cord.

In no way could I accept this, so I fell through an 18-foot scaffold while putting a roof on our house. I did a nice paratrooper landing on the brick patio. As I rolled backward from my feet to my buttocks, the bundle of shingles that I'd had on my shoulder while up on the scaffold fell on my head. The shingle bundle was followed very shortly by two pieces of the two-by-twelve board which had conveniently broken in order to let me fall through the scaffold. (I learned about time warp on the way down through the scaffold. It felt like it took several minutes to go from 18 feet in the air to the brick patio.)

The result of the accident was that the shingle bundle and planking fell on my head and pounded my head into my spine down to about the third and fourth thoracic vertebrae. In retrospect, I had put a dandy Energy Cyst into my upper thoracic spine.

I got osteopathic manipulation by two or three of my colleagues about 50 times with little or no relief. I had a constant pain in my upper thoracic spine and related muscles, [20] the scapulae, the shoulders and both arms. I felt like I wanted about 500 pounds of traction to pull on these vertebrae to decompress them. No one seemed able to help me.

I thought about Nogier's ideas in *Auriculotherapy* as I drove to the hospital one afternoon to make my rounds. (I had to fall through a scaffolding and almost kill myself in order to accept the idea that one might successfully treat the total body via the ear.) I took my left ear between my thumb and index finger. I started pressing on the cartilage in the areas where the cervical and upper thoracic vertebrae and soft tissue were represented. I found a place that really "hurt good" and pressed with my fingernail. As I did, my ear hurt more but my whole upper back and arm-shoulder pain syndrome started to ease up. My pain syndrome was enough to motivate me to do this ear pressure at least four or five times a day. The syndrome continued to improve and had nearly disappeared after about two weeks. (I suppose I should thank the scaffolding company for sending me a defective plank. Or

---

[20] In retrospect, my emotional status at that time was very conducive to retention of an Energy Cyst: I was angry, frustrated and having a number of marital problems.

perhaps I could thank whoever arranged this scenario. It seems to be more than a coincidence.)

Soon I was using ear acupuncture in conjunction with body acupuncture very successfully. Then I started to inject minuscule drops of Vitamin B12 into the addiction points of the ear in order to treat narcotics addicts. It worked beautifully to ease the withdrawal syndrome and reduce the desire for more drugs. This experience opened another world for me.

OPENING TO THE PSYCHIC

In the late '60s I was pretty sure that psychics, fortune tellers, healers and the like were all a bunch of con artists. (I was a little bit open on this subject, perhaps, but not much.) In about 1970, the real forces of the universe decided to run me through a series of experiences in order to open my mind to the reality of psychic phenomena. I was 38 years old, and at the time I was engaged in a rather acute general osteopathic medical and surgical practice: lots of heart attacks and strokes and trauma from the beaches were my daily fare.

I also had purchased a 200-seat restaurant and lounge. (All jazz musicians want to have their own club someday. I managed to do it. Whew, such a memory!) One evening my bartender/manager, Gordon, came to me and said, "Doc, you need to get a replacement for me." I asked why. (I'd thought Gordon was happy. As far as I knew we were good friends.)

Gordon said to me that he had just seen a psychic lady named Harriet in St. Petersburg. Harriet had told him that within three months he would take a new job at $25,000 per year salary, plus an expense account, plus a company Lincoln to drive. He would wear a suit and a tie every day. I hid my disbelief to some extent but not very well, I'm sure. Gordon had not completed high school. He was bright and experienced in the bar business—but what did an old psychic lady in St. Petersburg named Harriet know about how the world really works? (Boy, would I live to eat my words.) I promptly forgot the incident.

About a month later Gordon gave me two weeks notice. He had been offered a job by two land developers who had come by the club for a drink, talked with Gordon, liked his style and hired him right out from under me. He was to meet prospective real estate customers at the airport, show them the land development project and deliver them to the office for the sales pitch. For this work he would receive a $25,000 annual salary, an expense account, a Lincoln in which he was to chauffeur the potential buyers—and he had to wear a suit and tie every day at work.

This was some coincidence! I thought to myself, "It just goes to show you how psychics like Harriet get their reputation. Every once in a while they are right." I supposed that if you guessed enough you had to hit it right once in a while. What a fine rationalization!

Within a few months, my wife and my office nurse announced that they were going together to see Harriet for a "reading." When my wife went into Harriet's reading room, Harriet exclaimed, "Oh, you poor dear, your husband is in the hospital." Then Harriet calmed down and said, "It's okay, he's a doctor; he's seeing his patients." This was true. I had dropped our son at the YMCA to go swimming, went to the hospital to see patients and returned about 15 minutes before the swimming time was over. At 3:45 p.m., I went into the bowling alley bar next to the YMCA and ordered a glass of beer, which I didn't really want, because my stomach was a little upset. I drank the beer anyway and picked up our son a couple of minutes after 4 p.m.

My wife was with Harriet from 3 to 4 p.m. that day. At 3:50 p.m., my wife told me Harriet interrupted the reading to tell her how foolish I was to drink a glass of beer when I really didn't want it. When my wife told me about this I *knew* that Harriet was working some sort of scam and was having me followed. How the instant communication occurred between my tail and Harriet, I didn't know, but I sure didn't believe any old psychic could know that I drank a glass of beer that I didn't want at 10 minutes to 4 p.m. (Come to think of it, how would the tail know I didn't want it? But I didn't think of that at the time.) In retrospect, I can certainly see how far we reach to explain something logically that we don't want to believe.

The events with Gordon and my wife piqued my curiosity to the point that I decided to see Harriet myself. I called. A pleasant voice said, "Hello, my dear." Could this be the mysterious psychic? It sounded more like Betty Crocker or Mrs. Olsen. I asked for a consultation appointment the following Monday morning if that would be possible. Harriet said that it would be fine at 11 a.m. on Monday. I asked if she wanted my name. She said, "No, I don't need a name. I know you'll be here." I asked how she knew that. She said that knowing such things was what she did.

At 11 a.m. on Monday I arrived at the back steps of a pleasant, rather old but cheery frame house with lots of flowers in the yard. I was in paint-stained hobby jeans, moccasins and a tee shirt. I had driven my old Austin Healy Sprite. I was sure no one would ever guess that I was a doctor. I stood at the top of three wooden steps and rapped on the screen door. Looking through the screen I had a view of a very pleasant kitchen done in bright colors with yellow as the dominant. A plump, cherubic, white-haired, rosy-cheeked grandmotherly-type person came to the door. I said, "Good morning, I have an appointment at 11 a.m. Is Harriet here?"

The grandmotherly-type lady said, "Good morning my dear. I've been waiting for you. You're the osteopath. I have a sore shoulder and you can fix it." In a bind like this one I could not come up with a logical explanation for how she knew that I was an osteopath. I hadn't even given a first name when I made the appointment. I was temporarily disarmed. (It would get worse very quickly.)

Harriet invited me in and asked if I would fix her shoulder before our reading. She said there was plenty of time. She had planned lunch for both of us after the consultation was over. She sat on a kitchen chair, I stood behind her, somewhat at a loss about what to do. I began to palpate the spinous processes of the lower cervical and upper thoracic region.

She said very quickly, "Oh no, you needn't bother with all that; just put your hands on my shoulders." I did. I didn't question or object, I just cupped one hand over each shoulder. My left hand began to get warm. (This was the first time I had ever noticed such a happening.)

Harriet said, "Oh you poor dear, you don't have quite enough energy. Blue Belle, come and help him." Within a second—I swear to you—the pantry door flew open. Very quickly, my hand became uncomfortably hot. Harriet's shoulder was better right away. She had convinced me. There weren't any electronic bugging devices or private detectives that could do this. I turned 180 degrees; my belief system did an about-face.

Harriet and I became rather good friends after that first consultation. I went to see her on quite a few more Mondays for several consecutive weeks. We treated and consulted and had lunch together. Harriet answered any questions I asked.

During our first session she totally astonished me. She became a different old lady and spoke to me in German, which I could not understand. She reverted back to herself, Harriet, and told me that the German lady was Mary Wahl who had told me to keep my feet dry and warm where I was going. Mary Wahl was my paternal grandmother. I had only seen her a few times. She died when I was three. Mary Wahl was her maiden name. I knew this only because I had seen my father's birth certificate when he died. (I was 13 at that time.) Why would I need my feet warm and dry? I didn't know that I would be moving to Michigan in 1975, after I had lived 11 years in Florida.

Harriet told me not to worry about the book, it would be finished and be a big success. I hadn't even thought about CranioSacral Therapy as yet. I was into acupuncture to some extent. She also told me that two doctors were competing for my attention at that time. One was a brown-skinned Polynesian (who I assume was the acupuncturist) and the other was a tall Caucasian man named Henry White.

The name Henry White jogged my memory. While I was a Biochemistry Fellow in Kirksville, Missouri, I was given an old library storage room for my office. I went through hundreds of dusty old books which were stored there. One of these old books was a notebook dated 1901. This notebook contained the class notes of an osteopathic student named Henry White. I had really enjoyed reading those notes. After I finished, the notebook just wasn't there one day; I had always wondered where it went. I still don't know, but what a coincidence that Harriet would see a spirit guide named Henry White who wanted to direct me along a given path. At the time, I was doing about 20 acupuncture treatments a week. The Polynesian must have had the upper hand with them.

As we became friends, Harriet told me a few things that I'll share with you. She said that my education was one of the assignments she had to complete before she died. She told me that on a bad day her skills were merely telepathic and she could tell someone what they were thinking which would impress them satisfactorily. On a good day, she could connect with the spirit guides around a person. If the guides were nice she would let them use her body to communicate. If bad spirits came around, she just told them to "be gone," and they would leave because she wasn't afraid. She told me that life's scenarios are preconceived by the spirits before we are born. We can cooperate with the scenarios and have a relatively easy life or we can be obstinate and contrary and have a difficult life. It is really our individual choice.

Harriet said that a single soul can divide and be two or more incarnate humans in order to play out a scenario and learn a lesson. (This explained the population explosion to some extent.) Most souls don't really enjoy the earthly life; it is just something they have to do in order to advance.

During that first consultation Harriet also predicted, quite accurately, that we would move north into a house on a hill with water in the back but the move wouldn't be permanent. We moved to Michigan in July 1975 and bought a large brick house on a hill with a marsh out back. (Harriet sent me a few patients after we moved to Michigan where I had joined a university faculty. The patients from Harriet always said, "Harriet says you are the one who will fix me.")

Harriet astonished me one day when she told me that she was diabetic and gave herself insulin injections. I inquired as to how many calories she ate per day and how many units of insulin she took every day. She said it was different every day. She pushed my "regular doctor" button with that statement. I delivered my lecture on balancing the number of calories and the number of units of insulin with controlled exercise and so on. She just said, "Oh my dear, that sounds so complicated. I've been taking whatever dose of insulin that Blue Belle tells me to take every morning for about 25 years now." I acceded that Blue Belle knew more about diabetes management than I did. Harriet died recently in her mid-eighties. I'm sure she finished her assignments and the variable insulin dosage had little or nothing to do with her demise. Or perhaps, the insulin offered her the opportunity for transition from this incarnation at her convenience.

Harriet truly changed my life.

DOORWAY TO A WHOLE NEW LIFE

After acupuncture let me know how little I really knew about how bodies work, and after Harriet let me know that psychic phenomena and psychics are real, I must have become properly open because along came Delbert. He is the man many of my students have heard me describe as the person who gave me my first and irrefutable personal look at the craniosacral system as a semiclosed hydraulic system. The experience occurred in 1971.

I was called by Delbert's daughter who asked me to please stop by and see her father that morning on the way to the hospital. I had been the family doctor for Delbert's daughter, Sandy, her husband, Vinny, and their child, Raymond, for some time. (In fact, I had delivered Raymond.) I had never seen Delbert before. I did know that Delbert had been a coal miner for some years. I also knew that he had been retired from the coal mining occupation for about 10 years. He was supposed to have had some degree of black lung disease. He was a native of West Virginia.

I arrived at Delbert's home around 9 a.m. I was greeted by Delbert's daughter, Sandy, and his wife, Geneva. Delbert was on the living room floor. The place smelled of whiskey. There was vomit on the floor. There was partially digested and fresh blood in the vomitus. Delbert was only semiconscious and looked like "death warmed over," as my mother used to say. I was a little upset with Sandy because she hadn't mentioned to me that Delbert was an alcoholic, which was my immediate assessment. I checked Delbert's vital signs. His blood pressure was low, his heart rate was rapid. Who could tell how long or how much he had been bleeding in the stomach and perhaps the esophagus. If this were alcoholism, he was probably bleeding in the esophagus from varicose veins which usually develop from increased back pressure from the liver. If that were true, the life expectancy was really poor.

I decided to get him to the hospital by ambulance without wasting time. I tried to get Sandy or Geneva to tell me that Delbert was an excessive user of alcohol. Both denied it. They wouldn't have had much motivation to lie to me now, so maybe something else was wrong. They said he had drunk some whiskey that morning to ease the pain in his stomach. Then he vomited the whiskey. That was when Sandy called me and that was why the place reeked of booze. The ambulance arrived and we all left for the hospital.

The original diagnostic workup I did with Delbert revealed liver dysfunction. It also revealed cystic formation at multiple sites in both liver and brain. There was not, however, the generalized liver disease associated with alcoholism. The lungs, of course, confirmed black lung disease of ancient origin. The stomach demonstrated some active ulceration. The esophagus did not show varicosities, so apparently the fresh blood I saw in the vomitus was gastric in origin.

Now we had to discover the cause of the cysts and ulcer. Blood tests showed that Delbert was quite anemic, which was no real surprise. Finally, with liver biopsy and blood agglutination tests, we were able to trace the probable cause to a systemic infection by a fungus named Echinococcus. Delbert responded well enough to conservative medical treatment, and I discharged him from the hospital after about three weeks. Shortly after discharge he called me and said that the bottoms of his feet hurt so badly that he couldn't walk. I stopped by his home on the way to the hospital one morning. The soles of his feet were cracked, peeling and rather black in color. I had never seen nor heard of anything like this in my young career. I asked around the staff and got no helpful suggestions. The dermatologist I sent Delbert to was of no help.

Then the trek of referrals to the medical center at Gainesville, Florida, began. Next, he went to Duke University Medical School in Durham, North Carolina. Finally, he went to the Coal Miners Hospital in West Virginia. The answers we got from those institutions related mostly to central nervous system problems, pulmonary disease, liver dysfunction (which was mild by now) and some constitutional inadequacy. There were no answers concerning the problem with his feet, and Delbert wasn't complaining about anything but his feet.

After all of this, Sandy and Geneva prevailed upon me to hospitalize Delbert once more to see if I could find the answer. I was not optimistic. A new neuro-surgeon had just joined the staff. He had been in general practice for nine years, then he'd done a general surgical residency here in the United States. He then went to Japan for his neurosurgical training. He had some new and different ideas—at least they were new to me. I asked him to examine Delbert. He did and suggested that there might be a problem in the cervical area of the meninges. In Japan he had seen this cause dystrophic responses elsewhere in the body. The problem with the skin of the feet might be due to some form of dystrophy.

He suggested a cervical myelogram. (This was prior to CT scans, MRIs and ultrasound diagnostic techniques.) We had to put a radio-opaque dye in the subdural space. Then we wilted the x-ray table head down so that the dye—which was injected in the lumbar region and which was heavier than cerebrospinal fluid—would get into the cervical area. There we saw it—an epidural (outside of the dura mater) calcification about a centimeter in diameter and perhaps one-fifth of a centimeter thick covering the midline in the mid-cervical region.

When the neurosurgeon suggested that the cervical plaque could be causing the foot problem, I was quiet and decided to go along with his ideas. After all, we had no other worthwhile leads to follow. We decided that we had better get that plaque of calcium out of there before it created further problems which might affect the spinal cord and so on. I was a little surprised that a cervically located plaque on the outside of the dural membrane could cause the bottoms of the feet to become sore, turn black and peel off. But I was running out of ability to be surprised after my experiences with acupuncture and my good friend Harriet. I should have asked Harriet what was wrong with Delbert, but I didn't think of doing that until much later. In any case, we performed the surgical removal of the calcified plaque a few days after the myelogram.

In order to perform the surgery, Delbert was put in a sitting position, leaning forward in an anesthesia chair. This position gave us good access to the back of his neck. We used a midline incision. We removed the posterior parts of C4 vertebrae and opened a nice, round operative field. The external surface of the dura mater was exposed, and there was our calcified plaque staring us in the face. The neurosurgeon instructed me to hold the dural membrane very still with Allis clamps while he removed the plaque from the dural membrane without cutting or puncturing this tissue. It was at this time that I got a firsthand look at the moving membrane that was to become the boundary of the semiclosed hydraulic system which is now the cornerstone of the PressureStat model we developed to explain the physiological activity of the craniosacral system.

As I tried to hold this membrane still—rather unsuccessfully—I realized that it was moving, rhythmically, centralward into the operative site and then peripheralward toward the outside of the body through the operative site. Neither the neurosurgeon nor the anesthesiologist had ever noticed anything like this before. Both were a little impatient with my questions because the idea of surgery is to get in, do your job and get out. There is not much tolerance for wasting time. Despite their impatience, I managed to time this rhythmical activity at about eight cycles per minute. It was not in synchronization with the patient's breathing which was visible via the breathing bag in the anesthesia machine. It certainly was not synchronous with the heart action which was visible on the cardiac monitor. It was a rhythm none of us in the operating room had ever witnessed before.

I felt that I was the only one who cared at that time. I was puzzled a little as I watched the dural membrane moving in and out of the operative site, despite my efforts to hold it still. It seemed to me that about the only mechanism that could produce this effect would be a rhythmical rise and fall in fluid pressure on the other side of the membrane. This suggested to me that the dural membrane was involved in a hydraulic pumping system that I knew very little about.

It was the experience at Delbert's surgery that started me on a path of clinical and basic scientific research which ultimately led to the development of the concepts of CranioSacral Therapy, Energy Cysts, SomatoEmotional Release and all the rest. Delbert's feet returned to normal after the surgery. It took about two months for this to happen. Delbert and his Echinococcus really changed my life. Thank you, Delbert. (He died of lung cancer in 1981, after I had moved to Michigan State University. Perhaps he was sure by then that I was well on the way to my new life.)

ONE MAJOR STOP ALONG THE WAY

During sophomore year at osteopathic college, we were introduced to cranial osteopathy. This would have been in late 1959 or early 1960. There was one lecture by a visiting lecturer who represented the Cranial Academy. Very few of us took this lecture seriously because he talked about the rhythmical movement of skull bones. Most of us believed that this was nonsense. I thought no more about it.

Then came the experience with Delbert. I did not make the connection right away, but I continued to be mildly puzzled about that movement of the dural membrane that I had witnessed during Delbert's surgery. Some months after the surgery I came across a notice in the *Journal of the American Osteopathic Association* which invited the reader to a five-day course in cranial osteopathy. The claim was that participants would learn to feel the movement of skull bones and use this movement to treat various conditions related to impaired movement of these bones. I decided to attend the course because it might be related to what I had witnessed during Delbert's surgery. A most impressive review of the anatomy of the skull and sacrum was presented.

Then we moved to the examining tables where instructors would help us feel with our hands just what these lecturers had talked about. When Dr. Wales, my table instructor, put her hands on my head, it felt like Jell-O. I could feel all of these movements inside of my own head. Then she put her hand under my sacrum. The same thing happened. My pelvis turned to Jell-O. Both my skull and my pelvis were rhythmically moving. When it was my turn to put my hands on, it was as though I had been feeling this motion for years. I did not accept the explanations of why this movement was present, but I certainly could not deny that I was feeling it.

I went back to my practice. The first three severe and chronic headache patients who came in asking for acupuncture treatment responded beautifully to my crude application of cranial osteopathic technique. I took the bait and the hook was set. I used the techniques more and more with great success.

When the opportunity presented for me to join a research department at Michigan State University's College of Osteopathic Medicine, I jumped at the chance. I had the opportunity to begin to demystify cranial osteopathy and perhaps to understand the mechanisms of this system which we were later to name the craniosacral system.

PYRAMID POWER

Just before we moved to Michigan in June 1975, I had purchased a Plexiglas pyramid. I didn't much believe all the claims I had read for pyramid power but I thought I would try it out for myself. I hadn't tried it in Florida, but when we arrived in Michigan I set the pyramid on top of a bookshelf in the breezeway between our house and garage. (The breezeway was a wooden structure with minimal electrical wiring.) I aligned the pyramid up to magnetic north and south and put a fresh daisy from the yard on the pedestal under the Plexiglas pyramid. I forgot about it for over a year. I was rearranging my books one day and I noticed the daisy in the pyramid. It seemed in perfect condition. I took it out from under the pyramid and it was very hard as though petrified. It was not brittle enough to be fragile, but it was very hard. I set the daisy on the window sill in the kitchen. Within 48 hours the petals were wilted and some had fallen off. It was now a typical wilted, unwatered cut flower. (Since I have been back in Florida I have tried to replicate this observation without any success. I suspect there is too much electrical pollution in my office.)

After the daisy experiment, we started putting the pyramid on our heads, on our sore knees, etc. We never really got serious about experimenting with it, but we did see the following:

1. A pyramid over a sore knee seemed to focus and intensify the pain for about 10 minutes, then the pain went away. (One particular sore knee was a bruise on my left kneecap from a fall on the ice.)

2. When I put the pyramid on my head I felt a cooling sensation on the top of my head which was rather pleasant. I felt as though I were in an air ventilation system with fresh cool air going up the sides of my cranial vault to the top. (I felt if I remained that way I would become a cone—or rather a pyramid—head).

3. When my wife put the pyramid on her head she got a headache almost immediately and became quite agitated. (I think we are from different planets.)

4. The pyramid sensations could be increased and decreased by rotating my body, with the pyramid on my head, in relation to the magnetic north and south poles.

We also built an eight-foot-per-side pyramid in the garden. We had about a half-acre vegetable garden. The pyramid seemed to accelerate the growth of the foliage, but it did not seem to affect the size of the underground tubers. For example, our spinach grew perhaps 50 percent larger and more quickly under the pyramid. Our turnips seemed the same as those not under the pyramid, although the tops grew more. We abandoned the pyramid in the garden because the weeds also were much hardier and grew more quickly under the pyramid. (Perhaps the pyramid and I differ in opinion as to the definition of the weed. Since then, I have been informed by a nursery owner that a weed is anything you don't plant.)

In summary, the pyramid certainly has an effect, and it is a powerful effect at that. I don't know how to use it effectively. Our observations with personal use demonstrate to me that "One man's meat is another man's poison." I think we should respect the pyramid a great deal and be very careful about how we use it. I wouldn't want to be petrified like my daisy. (I wondered if this energy could be related to the energy that fused the tissue to the acupuncture needle or if they are two separate systems, perhaps two separate methods of focusing the same energy.)

HANDS-ON ENERGY BECOMES APPARENT

We had just arrived at our new home in East Lansing, Michigan. We had moved ourselves, so there was a caravan of two passenger cars and one large rent-a-truck. This was the family and all of our belongings. While we were unloading the furniture from the truck, our realtor, Tomie, came by. She was a very nice lady who had been very accommodating in helping us purchase the house we were moving into. (She had even given us a short-term loan to make the down payment on time.) To make a long story short, when she asked if I would treat her right shoulder as soon as my treatment table was unloaded, I said "yes," even though I wasn't really in the mood after a couple of hours of furniture moving and a two-day drive in a truck. She had waited around for me to unload the table, so what could I do? She had me.

We went into the room that was to be a sort of study. (Actually, it was the breezeway between the house and garage where I later placed my pyramid.) We set up the portable treatment table and she sat on it. I stood behind her. I cupped my hands over her shoulders much as I had done for Harriet the psychic who expanded my mind a couple of years before.

Within seconds I could feel a line of heat develop in Tomie's right shoulder. It was precisely where the triple heater meridian courses over the shoulder (although the fact did not dawn on me at the time.) This line of heat got hotter and hotter. I was not thinking much; I was very tired and sort of coasting. I stood behind Tomie for perhaps 15 minutes as the line of heat that traversed her right shoulder became uncomfortably hot. The heat built to a crescendo which was very hot. I felt a lot of pain and burning across the palm of my hand where it approximated the line of heat. This discomfort lasted a minute or so. Tomie did some heavy breathing and perspiring. Suddenly everything got quiet. She smiled and said the pain was gone. My hand felt better. The treatment was obviously over. I didn't have the slightest idea what I had done to facilitate the therapeutic response, but I knew that I would try it again as soon as I had the chance.

I carried a red line across my palm for three days after this treatment. This line across my palm was about a half-inch wide and traveled from the thenar eminence to the base of the fifth finger. It felt like a sunburn, and it didn't really bother me unless something contacted it; then it gave me a burning sensation. What had happened? In retrospect, I think I opened my first acupuncture meridian by hand. It was a good time to have this experience because my fatigue had taken my left brain pretty much out of the way.

Tomie's shoulder never gave her another problem after that treatment experience. That occurred in June 1975. I saw her regularly both as a patient and socially until we left Michigan in December 1982. In fact, Tomie has visited with us in Florida over Christmas holidays on three occasions since then. Still, there has been no right shoulder pain recurrence.

PULLING ENERGY THROUGH THE MERIDIA OF ACUPUNCTURE

Tomie's daughter, Sandy, was really the next person to give me another lesson in the hands-on opening of acupuncture meridia. This occurred in the fall of 1975. Sandy lived in Fort Lauderdale, Florida. She had awakened one Sunday morning minus the use of her left arm. She had seen a neurologist and was doing physiotherapy at his recommendation. The arm and shoulder were painful and dysfunctional. She was using an arm sling and was not getting any better. Sandy was an airline stewardess and could fly up to Michigan if I would see her. All of this came to me via her mother, Tomie.

Sandy came to Michigan and I saw her each weekday over a two-week period. By this time, I was into Kirlian photography. The pictures of her fingers showed a much smaller energy output from the left hand than from the right. I did some acupuncture to reduce the pain. This was reasonably successful in reducing the pain, but it did not equalize the Kirlian photographs between her two hands when I redid them after each treatment. Nor did it restore the strength to the left arm and hand. Sandy did not have enough strength to hold a full cup of water with her left hand. Both the oppositional strength of thumb and fingers as well as the wrist strength were very much reduced.

The Fort Lauderdale neurologist had not come up with a firm diagnosis. After a couple of symptom-reducing acupuncture treatments, I did some structural corrections to the cervical and upper thoracic vertebra and to the ribs. I didn't know anything about arcing as yet.

I found myself wondering if the hands-on energy work would be of any help. I held her left hand with my left hand in a handshake grip. Her hand felt cold and relatively lifeless. I put my right hand around her wrist and just thought about the hand and wrist warming, vitalizing and getting strong. Sure enough, some warming occurred. Then I got a sense that fluid or something was beginning to flow in the hand and wrist. I didn't say anything, nor did Sandy. We just sat for about five minutes, both of us feeling the changes.

Suddenly it dawned on me that I could feel the acupuncture meridia as they passed through her wrist. I concentrated on each meridian individually. It seemed that the greatest change and flow of fluid was in the volar wrist region where the pericardial (circulation-sex) meridian conducts energy (chi). This meridian takes origin in the pericardium of the chest and flows to its termination on the end of the third finger. I thought it was a good meridian to provide revitalization to the arm and hand.

I began to urge the meridian mentally to flow and I visualized an open connection between it and the triple heater meridian which returns chi energy centralward to the body. This seemed to work. Either consciously or nonconsciously, Sandy began to experiment with her hand. She began to move her fingers and tighten and loosen her grip. The warmth in her hand was improving quite remarkably.

I let my hands think for themselves. (This was before I knew they had more intelligence than my head.). My hands, both of them, went to Sandy's upper arm. They fashioned a ring around her upper arm just below the axilla. I had my thumb tips touching on one side and my middle fingertips touching on the other side of the arm. Gradually, I began to "pull" energy from her shoulder into her arm as though my hands were magnetic. As this energy got to her arm at the level of my hands (still forming the ring around her arm), I slowly moved my hand-formed ring-magnet distalward, carrying the sense of vitalization and energy with me. If I moved too fast, I lost contact with whatever it was I was pulling with me. (I rationalized that the pericardial, heart and lung acupuncture meridians all conduct energy and vitalization away from the body, so I worked with these meridia to open them. The large intestine, triple heater and small intestinal meridia all conduct proximally—from hand to trunk—therefore I worked against them. I thought that would be okay, however, because I would sort of "back flush" these latter three meridia.) In any case, I kept the ring that I had formed with my hands intact and moved very slowly and painstakingly distalward along the upper arm, being very careful to bring the sense of vitalization with me. I passed the elbow without difficulty; I slowly moved my hands (still forming the ring-magnet) down the forearm to the wrist.

At the wrist my hands decided to change their position. I really felt like I was a privileged spectator to what my hands were doing. My right hand arranged itself longitudinally so that it covered the dorsum of Sandy's proximal phalanges, hand and wrist. My left hand did the same thing on her volar surface. I had make a sandwich with her hand as the meat (or for the vegetarian, the peanut butter) and my two hands were the two pieces of bread. The middle fingers of my two hands paralleled the Triple Heater and pericardial meridia. I began to pull distally (in my mind's eye) with my left hand on the volar surface of Sandy's hand. I pushed proximally (again in my mind's eye) with my right hand on the dorsal surface of Sandy's hand. There was some perceived resistance for awhile. Suddenly, very suddenly, there was an opening and a softening and a flowing and everything good that you can think of. Immediately after what I would now call a "release," Sandy smiled. I took my hands away and she felt "normal."

I redid the Kirlian photographs: her hands were close to equal. I shot my own fingers as well and there was corona energy going all over the place.

This took place on Friday, at the end of the first week. I continued to see the patient daily during the second week but this was more for me than it was for her arm and hand. She was fine and remained fine. (I have no idea what caused this to happen to Sandy. Perhaps it occurred because I needed to learn another lesson. Thank you, Sandy.)

OUR OWN BODIES ARE THE BEST LABORATORIES

It was the fall of 1978. Our research had been going quite successfully at Michigan State University. The concepts of PressureStat Model, Energy Cyst, Direction of Energy and SomatoEmotional Release were all falling pretty well into place.

I was at home one day pruning some rather large shrubs. I trimmed a branch and the cut end rebounded directly into the cornea of my left eye. The pain was phenomenal: I experienced the distribution of the trigeminal nerve and its connections with the reticular alarm system. It took all I could do to keep from yelling hysterically and running around the yard like a maniac. I reasoned with myself and felt a little more stable and objective about the situation. I opened my injured left eye. Everything was a total blur. I could see light, but I was sure that I had damaged the cornea. I'd never before had a sensation like this.

Finally, I went into the house and asked my wife to look at my eye. She said there was a big "dent in the shape of a 'Y' laying on its side" that went across my pupil. Suddenly I was in touch with how much I did not want to damage my cornea and impair vision. I thought about seeing an ophthalmologist, going to the emergency room—it all seemed like too much to think about. I knew what they would do and I did not want that.

Suddenly I heard myself say, "Hey, dipsh _ _, you teach the V-spread all the time. If you really believe in it, why not try it on yourself?" I went into the bedroom and lay down on the bed. I looked at my watch. The time was 1:50 p.m. I made a "V" of my left index and middle fingers with the eyeball between the proximal phalanges of the two fingers (in the crotch of the "V"). I experimented for a position around the back of my head which felt right for my sending fingers. That position turned out to be just below the posterior occipital protuberance on the midline. I used my index, middle and ring fingers to send energy from this locus through my left eyeball. After a minute or two I could feel energy building. My eyeball began pulsating. It hurt a lot. It seemed like forever. I thought it probably wouldn't work. The eye pain got worse but I kept on with the V-spread, "just because." All of a sudden there was a "pop" in my eyeball—which I was sure could be heard in the other room. Immediately after the "pop" occurred, the pain left. The blurred vision cleared. My anxiety disappeared. I was filled with elation. It had worked! My eye was okay.

I went into the living room and found my wife. She had not heard the "pop" but she said that the dent in my cornea was gone.

My confidence in energy direction as a therapeutic modality—and as a real phenomenon—was bolstered several hundred percent. I thanked the bush for cooperating. I thank whoever composes these scenarios when they seem appropriate. I was a different person after this experience. I could really teach the direction of energy with no holds barred. What a beautiful experience!

UNDERSTANDING MY BODY AND ITS RESPONSES

I had just returned from a 10-week journey in Europe and Israel. I was really tired. I had been living out of a suitcase for two and a half months, teaching, setting up two clinical research projects and demonstrating techniques. The stress had definitely taken its toll. The flight from Tel Aviv's Ben Gurion Airport to Detroit was long; it took 27 hours. Then we had to drive from Detroit to East Lansing. Our luggage had been lost but it was good to be home, with or without it.

On the flight between New York and Detroit I began to feel my throat getting sore, and my chest began to tighten up. I felt it must have been the air conditioning on the plane and maybe the positive ionic charge that is created by the friction of air on the fuselage. I developed a cough after we arrived home and it was persistent. I was tired and suffered jet lag, so I was not surprised to feel exhausted. I started on heavy doses of multivitamins and tried to get some rest.

I didn't get much better or much worse for a week. The cough and sore throat persisted and it hurt to breathe. My trachea and bronchial tubes seemed raw and virtually resented the passage of air. I couldn't take a deep breath. I hurt all over.

One evening I started to cough and couldn't get a breath. It hurt from my diaphragm to my mouth, but I couldn't stop coughing and I couldn't inhale; I didn't have time between coughs. Suddenly, it didn't matter. Then nothingness. The next thing I heard was my wife calling my name somewhat frantically.

I came awake quickly and felt much better—no pain. I could breathe and I didn't give a darn about anything. I thought my wife was unduly upset but I guess she had a right to be upset. She had seen me cough and cough then suddenly slump forward in the chair and stop breathing, and she had pounded on my chest with her fist. My body must have released a dose of endorphin or some such thing because I felt fine. It must be the same sensation that makes people euphoric during severe pain or when death is eminent. As a physician, I had seen it happen many times.

In any case, I became aware that certain parts of my lungs would not fill with air, that I was wheezing loudly enough to be heard across the room and that if I attempted any exertion I became hypoxic. I was aware of my heart activity and of every little intercostal muscle working to rhythmically increase and decrease the volume of my thoracic cage. I was, indeed, a very detached observer of my own circumstance. Oddly, this attitude of detachment and the great reduction in pain sensitivity persisted for more than two weeks, the approximate time I required to regain some of my health.

During the period immediately following the episode of unconsciousness, it seemed to me that death and I had been introduced. It didn't feel at all bad and I was perfectly willing to allow death to take me if it were meant to be. I felt absolutely no fear. The only thing I was sure of was that I did not wish to take steps to aid death in taking me, that I would put forth a good effort and abide by the outcome without any regret. I also was sure, somehow, that I would be fighting unfairly if I took any antibiotic or allowed myself to be hospitalized. I didn't want to have my breathing done for me nor to be artificially oxygenated nor anything else. I wanted to see what my body/mind/spirit complex could do. I had developed a strong belief that given common sense support, manipulative treatment and some pampering, the human body can best survive serious encounters with pathogenic forces and be stronger for having met those challenges.

(I had been smoking one to two packs of cigarettes daily for about 25 years—with one three-year respite in the middle. After the above episode, I lost all desire and need to smoke. This has not returned and I have had no tobacco since the experience, more than 14 years ago.)

As fate would have it, I was now to have the opportunity to compare various approaches by three osteopathic physicians, all using their hands to do osteopathic manipulative therapy. I was treated every day by one or another. Each used quite different techniques.

Harold is a British osteopath who arrived from London with his wife to spend four days visiting with us. Their arrival was just four days after my introduction to death. Upon hearing my wheezing and observing my sallow color, Harold offered to treat me osteopathically. He treated me once or twice daily for four days. (He was concerned about overtreatment but opted to do so with my encouragement.)

Harold does, almost exclusively, what the British call "functional technique" although he is well acquainted with various direct techniques such as thrust, articulatory and muscle energy. He is a graduate of and instructor at the European School of Osteopathy. Harold's approach was simply to place his hand over an area of tissue abnormality, be it on the front or back of the thorax. Sometimes he used two hands, one on the area of involvement and the other on top of the head (monitoring parietal bone motion). Or he might place the second hand elsewhere on the thorax. (There was little consistency in the placement of the second hand.) As he held the treating hand over the selected area of involvement, the following occurred:

1.   My skin, where it was in contact with his hand, became very hot, then the heat moved deeper into my body and viscera as well as Harold's treating hand—almost uncomfortably so. As the heating process was going on over a period of several minutes, I felt increasing quantities of inherent body motion at the area of involvement. This was frequently a revolving or circumduction type of motion around a minimally moving pivot point deep in the tissues.

As the heat became more apparent, the pivot point of minimal motion (which I interpret to be an area of restriction) seemed to dissolve so that the treated region began to move more in concert with the rest of the thorax. All of these motions referred to are rhythmical and synchronous with craniosacral motion.

2.   As the motion of the treated region came into concert with the rest of the thorax, I began to wheeze louder and louder with each breath.

3.   Ultimately and in only a few minutes, I began to cough harder and harder, producing sputum, so this was very satisfying: Prior to and between these treatments, my coughing was uncontrollable, tight and not productive. (As the treatment progressed, the sputum, which started as yellow and thick, became white and frothy.)

4.   Dyspnea was greatly relieved with each treatment and although regression occurred between treatments, it did not regress to the same starting point each time. (One might say that I took three giant steps forward during each treatment and, perhaps, two giant steps backward between treatments.)

I could literally feel my body fighting the infection. With the development of this awareness I was able to focus my attention on specific visceral areas that seemed tight and achieve some minor therapeutic successes by my own effort. It amazed me that as my own body awareness improved, I could tell precisely where the foci of major physiological difficulty were located. Harold, without any prompting from me, treated exactly those areas.

Overall, I must say that Harold's treatment was very powerful and effective in terms of my own body response to its application. I am very suspicious that Harold's brand of osteopathic treatment kept me out of the hospital or perhaps kept me alive, depending upon which would have come first. Realistically, I am sure he helped strengthen my body defenses a great deal and at the very least shortened my illness, made it less severe and obviated the need for antibiotic and/or other suppressive medical care.

After Harold's departure I was treated daily by Sister Anne, a student at Michigan State University's College of Osteopathic Medicine and a longtime dear friend. She applied the same treatment approach as Harold with similar although somewhat lesser apparent effect.

Sister Anne treated me daily for about one week after Harold left. I tried very hard to make it a proper learning experience for her. Initially, she was not at all sure that she could use Harold's techniques successfully, but she did try and, as I said, the results were similar if somewhat less dramatic. Her hands did not get as hot; my viscera did not get as hot; and I didn't cough as effectively, but I did hold my own and showed some improvement during this week of the illness. (In retrospect I think she was not as effective because she treated with some self-doubt.)

Then Seldon, an osteopath from Ohio, arrived. He used some direct thrust technique on specific paravertebral lesions. I could discern no visceral effect or improvement in my ability to breathe from these techniques, although they were successful in correcting somatic dysfunction of the ribs, thoracic and cervical vertebrae. He also used some general rib-raising techniques which offered immediate improvement in my dyspnea, but it was very general and did not feel as though the loci of difficulty were being affected as they had been with Harold's and Sister Anne's work.

The most effective thing Seldon did, from my point of view, was the lymphatic pump. He used my feet as levers and pumped for prolonged periods of time while I lay supine. We also found that when I held my breath for prolonged periods, the effect of this treatment was facilitated. The sequence of events I experienced during the application of the lymphatic pump was as follows:

1. A rhythmical motion began through the whole body in time with the pumping technique. This body response required three to five minutes to develop.

2. Gradually, I could feel a gliding motion developing between the skin of my posterior thorax—which was directly in contact with the table—and the posterior osseous structures of the thoracic cage. (I suspect that a great deal of the beneficial effect was derived from the stimulation of reflex areas located in the posterior thoracic fascia. It was during these treatments that we discovered that respiratory assistance greatly enhanced the therapeutic effect.)

3. With continuation of the lymphatic pump technique, I began to feel as though the tissues deep in the osseous structures of the posterior thorax e.g. fascia, pleura and lungs began to soften and move/glide independently of one another.

4. As the lymphatic pumping continued, I began to wheeze very deeply and more and more loudly. (From the sound of my breathing it was apparent that abnormal and viscous secretions were thinning or liquefying.)

5. After about 30 seconds of wheezing I would typically begin to cough. The cough was productive of large quantities of yellow sputum coming from very deep in my respiratory tree. This was followed by some improvement of dyspnea.

Seldon was in town for two days, and we repeated the treatment three times during that period. Each time, my physiological response was similar: The sputum became more white and frothy and less yellow with successive treatments. Dyspnea was greatly improved by the series of treatments given by Seldon. I feel that the lymphatic pump was extremely effective in my case.

Following Seldon's departure I became convinced that my body was winning the war with the pathogens. Sister Anne now treated me daily with the lymphatic pump technique. The treatment continued to be effective and my lungs seemed fairly well cleaned out a few days after Seldon left. Sister Anne also made some structural corrections as they seemed indicated but none seemed to have any immediate effect upon my respiratory function. (Structural corrections probably do favorably effect viscera, but the relationship was not as directly apparent to me as a patient.)

Now, I found my chest tightening up and I began coughing when I had to inhale irritants such as other people's cigarette smoke and the like. When I left those spaces and got into some clean air space my chest loosened very quickly and I was okay. My only sputum now was white and frothy.

I now felt well enough to decide to return to work part time. I decided that since the distance from home to office was approximately three miles, I would walk it every morning and this would aid in my recovery. About one-half mile into the walk I would consistently begin to wheeze. I would continue walking (at a rate of three to four miles per hour). The wheeze always became louder until I began to cough and produce sputum. Occasionally the sputum was yellow but more often it was white and frothy. (The walk had a similar therapeutic physiological effect to that which was obtained by Seldon with his lymphatic pump. The effect was not as specific as that obtained by Harold with his functional technique.)

After four or five days, the wheezing and coughing began to occur later in the walk (one to one and a half miles); it lasted for a shorter duration and ultimately disappeared. It is interesting to note that I could always walk through the wheezing and coughing episodes and feel better overall after the coughing stopped than I had before it started. (Six weeks later I was still walking to and from work at a rate of four miles per hour, with absolutely no coughing for about four weeks.)

This experience is similar to one recounted by a good friend, Dick MacDonald, D.O. Dick is a serious runner. He has told me that on several occasions if he became ill he would start running. After he ran for awhile, the subjective symptoms would worsen, but if he kept on running they would improve. He states that he always feels better by the end of the run. He has experienced this phenomenon on several occasions with sore throats and respiratory infections.

My own experience with this illness and walking would seem to confirm Dick's experience. I feel sure, through personal experience, that walking and lymphatic pumping serve to mobilize body fluids containing powerful defense mechanisms. It may be that pathogens have a much easier time when body fluids are in a state of relative immobility. It may also be that illness is perpetuated by sympathetic hypertonus—which may be related to reduced mobility of body fluids—and that exercise, be it active (as in walking) or passive (as in lymphatic pumping) results in the reduction of sympathetic nervous system tonus.

As I write this [in the summer of 1989], I have experienced little or no desire to resume cigarette smoking. In fact, I am repulsed by smoke and the odor of cigarettes.

I hope this subjective review of my experiences with various manipulative techniques proves instructive. I know the experience was a very valuable one for me. I do not recommend illness as a learning device to all of you, but I must say that experience is a most effective teacher. I'm sure it served its purpose.

I have used techniques similar to the functional approach employed by Harold for some years now. I have seen the results in patients but have always questioned (deep down in the scientific part of my soul) exactly what was going on. Any skepticism once held toward this approach has been completely dispelled by this experience. The functional approach was, by far, the most effective, most specific and least trying from my point of view as a patient. The next most effective treatment was the supine position foot lever lymphatic pump with respiratory assistance as applied by Seldon. Walking was almost comparable but a little less effective than the lymphatic pump.

MY EXPERIENCE WITH CO_2 - O_2 INHALATION

During a two-day seminar in February 1980 at the CME Center in Pontiac, Michigan, Dr. June MacRae and I arranged to do some preliminary investigation into the effects of CO_2 inhalation upon the function of the craniosacral system. A Dr. Meduna at the University of Illinois had developed a therapy wherein patients inhaled a mixture of 20 to 30 percent carbon dioxide in oxygen. It was used for neuroses and various dysfunctions such as stuttering and nervous tics. The question of a possible relationship between his approach and CranioSacral Therapy occurred to me while I was reading Dr. Meduna's case histories. The described clinical courses of many of my craniosacrally-treated patients seemed to parallel the clinical courses of many of his CO_2 - O_2-treated patients. The obvious question was, "Does CO_2 - O_2 inhalation affect the craniosacral system and its function?"

In order to explore this question, it initially seemed reasonable to rely upon my subjective impression of craniosacral system events—as transmitted through my hands from the subjects during the course of several CO_2 - O_2 mixture inhalations. After manually monitoring the craniosacral system function of five different subjects, I was satisfied that the inhalation of CO_2 - O_2 mixture did (in all five cases) result in spontaneous release of craniosacral system restrictions. There was also a marked increase in craniosacral amplitude with less membranous resistance to motion.

The gas mixture in these initial trials was 30 percent CO_2 with 70 percent O_2 administered by mask and breathing bag in a closed ventilatory system. Most subjects took three to five inhalations of the gas mixture followed by a rest of about three to four minutes. We repeated this cycle about 10 times for each subject. (One subject did take 15 deep breaths on one occasion. He had previous experience with CO_2 - O_2 inhalation.)

My impression while monitoring these subjects during CO_2 - O_2 inhalation was that progressive craniosacral system corrections were accomplished as the sets of inhalations were repeated for each person i.e., usually the amplitude of craniosacral system motion markedly increased during the first and second set of inhalations; during rest periods the amplitude would decrease again. The craniosacral system seemed progressively more relaxed and easy in its motion after each set of inhalations. After two or three rest periods the craniosacral system began to produce its own Still Points. These occurrences were followed by marked and significant releases of membranous restriction with spontaneous correction of a variety of motion distortions. I am convinced that similar corrections might have taken several minutes, if not hours, of treatment time to achieve by the manual approach. The observation begs further careful investigation.

Since I was considering the use of the combination of CO_2 - O_2 inhalation with manual CranioSacral Therapy for brain dysfunctioning children, the sixth subject had to be me. I would not apply the CO_2 - O_2 treatment in these cases without first experiencing it.

This is how it felt to me: The first inhalation of CO_2 - O_2 gas mixture seemed generally acceptable to my body. Exhalation was difficult somehow. The second inhalation was somewhat tentative but was achievable. The second exhalation was not possible at first, my chest would not allow it. I finally exhaled a little bit. The third inhalation volume was, therefore, significantly reduced since the second exhalation was not complete. After the third inhalation the mask was removed. I had great difficulty fully exhaling, but what a relief to have that mask off my face!

During my first CO_2 - O_2 breathing experience, we did four mask sets of three inhalations each. I had seen an orange background with white polka dots as a visual hallucination. I vividly recalled a near-drowning incident which had occurred when I was about 10 years old. I was at Olsen's Beach in St. Clair Shores, Michigan. I was there with my friend Gordon, a better swimmer than I. There were many people swimming and we decided to swim out to the end of the dock where the water was about six or eight feet deep. I couldn't make it and was floundering, but no one paid any attention because they all thought I could swim. The water was very brown and murky. My reflexes were all trying to make me exhale but I was underwater and knew that if I exhaled I would have to inhale and then I would drown. I vividly recalled my respiratory system bucking, trying to stop me from exhaling—just as was happening during the CO_2 - O_2 inhalations. Finally, Gordon saw my plight and yelled for help. Some larger boys pulled me out of the water, laid me on my stomach on the dock and proceeded to further prevent me from breathing by awkwardly applying artificial respiration, or so it seemed. I recalled them pushing the air out of my lungs while I was trying to take air in—exactly the same feeling I had during the CO_2 - O_2 inhalations.

I also clearly remembered the ether anesthesia for my tonsillectomy at age 4. I remembered that the doctor said that he was pouring water on the mask. That "water" smelled terrible. I fought as hard as I could. I really couldn't breathe. I wondered why they wanted to kill me. Where was my mother and even more significantly, where was my father? I was so scared.

The night of the CO_2 - O_2 inhalation I had very clear dreams of the drowning incident. Then I dreamed that I removed my sternal plate, as one would during an autopsy, and threw it away. I felt much lighter but more vulnerable. I had mixed feelings. I did not want to completely discard my sternum. It was my defense, my armor. I took it out and put it back several times. I don't know where my sternum was when I awakened at 5:30 a.m.

A few days later, back in my office in East Lansing, I had a strong desire to inhale more CO_2 - O_2. It was as though something needed to go to completion. I called Dr. MacRae and she agreed to work further with me. This time my breathing was better but I still bucked a lot and had difficulty with exhalation. I then recalled being hit in the solar plexus and not being able to breathe. My thoracic cage just wouldn't move. It was my first year playing high school football. I was lying on the ground. The coach looked at me rather disdainfully and commented that I was okay. "Just had the wind knocked out of you." I was mortified. I couldn't move for what seemed like hours. I'm sure the memory was a CO_2 - O_2-induced SomatoEmotional Release.

After re-experiencing this memory I did better with the CO_2 - O_2 but still had some difficulty with full exhalation. Dr. MacRae suggested that we add just one inhalation in a set to obtain better relaxation. It helped and I could inhale deeper and exhale more fully because I knew my next breath would be without the mask. I felt safer and in control.

After a deep inhalation I felt like I had a rod in my spine. My body felt fairly relaxed around this rod. Dr. MacRae suggested this rod sensation was symbolic that I was accepting too much responsibility for others. After some conversation, she helped me realize that the only one who can make me accept the responsibility for others is me. She suggested that, in fact, God was ultimately responsible for everyone. If I was not God I need not allow others to be dependent upon me. I then realized that I ask for this dependency. When I get what I ask for, I rebel against it because it gets too heavy. This is probably a syndrome shared by many physicians.

I envisioned a lead bar placed diagonally across my sternum after the second to last inhalation of CO_2 - O_2 that day. That night I dreamed a lot and realized that several events had created a weight on my chest. The events I dreamed of were as follows:

1.   At the time of my father's death, I had just turned 13 years of age. I was awakened from a sound sleep by my mother calling me. My father, whom I loved dearly, was lying on the couch and my mother was rubbing his chest. She told me to telephone Dr. Cross. I could not discriminate the letters in the phone directory; I had lost my ability to read. In a panic, Mother screamed at me and left my father to come and call the doctor herself. My father was dead when the fire department arrived. I was totally confused. I accepted responsibility for my father's death. I loved him so much. It was my fault that he died that night.

2.   At my father's funeral I was sobbing uncontrollably and could not get my breath; it felt just like my experience with the CO_2 - O_2 inhalations.

3.   Someone told me after the funeral that I was now the man of the family. I was responsible for taking care of my mother. I didn't remember the face of the person but I could hear his voice. I felt very afraid and inadequate.

4.   I questioned the minister at our church as to why my father was taken by this "loving God." The minister lost patience with my questions and told me to go away and not return to the church until I was able to restore my faith in God and accept his works. I never went back.

All of these factors became clear in my dreams that night—after this further work with the CO_2 - O_2 inhalations. By morning it was clear to me that I accept responsibility and I solicit dependency. When it gets too heavy, I rebel. The dependent people may then become angry and hurt by my refusal to continue to accept their dependence. Then I feel guilty about that. Perhaps, I thought, I play God because I will be better at it than the God who so cruelly took my father. All of this had made my anterior thoracic cage immobile so that I couldn't breathe properly.

It was over. When I walked to work that morning, my ribs were snapping and cracking with pleasure as they mobilized. I was breathing deeply like a child. I had found a new toy, breath. I began to run without getting short of breath. I had been short-winded since I was a teenager. I had given up basketball and did not go out for track because of this short-windedness. Instead I played football, hockey and lifted weights. It is wondrous the way events shape our lives. Had I not developed the neurotic pattern now clear to me, I probably would not be an osteopathic physician today. I probably would not be considering the effect of CO_2 - O_2 inhalation upon the craniosacral system. Thank you again, whoever you are.

REINCARNATION? WHAT NEXT?

In July 1978, a French osteopath, Jean-Pierre Barral, told me that I had some spasm of the left ureter. In July 1979, he told me the same thing. The closest I could come to agreeing with him was a recurrent condition of shingles that occurred only when I was under a lot of stress and which I controlled by self acupuncture. (It was at the level of the eighth intercostal nerve on the left and pretty well followed this nerve's distribution.)

In January 1980 Jean-Pierre Barral was visiting us in Michigan. He examined me "off the body" as he does. He told me there was an abnormal heat pattern over my upper left abdominal quadrant and over the left inferior costal region. He uses heat or energy patterns to determine how old the person was when the injury or illness occurred; he only needs to know the subject's current age. Jean-Pierre moved his hands about for a few minutes. His face took on an expression of disbelief. His voice developed a tone of marked astonishment. He finally said, "John, this is an injury from 140 years ago." (That would be the year 1840.)

As he spoke, I remembered an experience prior to our move to Michigan in 1975. A friend and I were playing around with hypnoregression. As the subject, I had seen myself as a black male slave in Charleston, South Carolina. I had decided to run away, ran for a day and hid the first night in a farmer's barn. He found me asleep in his barn early the next morning. I came awake suddenly with him standing over me, about to plunge a pitchfork into my body. I died of fright before he stabbed me in the upper left abdomen and lower left thorax. As I died, I flew up above and watched the anger of the farmer as he plunged the pitchfork into my vacated body. I laughed at him derisively.

In retrospect, I reconsider my behavior at the time of this death. My attitude of derision was deplorable. I see again the angry farmer, so controlled and driven by his emotions, prejudices and hatred acting so inhumanely against another human being. I recalled this incident as Dr. Barral worked with me non-verbally. Suddenly, I felt total compassion for the farmer. (I hope that some time I can see him again and help him as I may be able. He needs to shed himself of his negative emotion. Perhaps we have met again since 1840?)

Thank you, Jean-Pierre. Can it be that we carry trauma from one life to another? Since this experience, I believe we do. I also feel sure we carry these traumas with us when the circumstances of death reflect an unacceptable resolution. My attitude of derision as the farmer stabbed me with the pitchfork was an unacceptable end to that lifetime. I understand that now and the symptoms are no longer with me.

Since Jean-Pierre's evaluation and my resolution of this "experience," I have had no further recurrence of my shingles. He no longer sees my ureter as a problem. At least he hasn't mentioned it lately.

ANOTHER INSIGHT

During the latter part of April 1980 I felt a powerful restlessness and dissatisfaction building up inside of me. In early May I went to Crystal River, Florida, to participate in the presentation of a seminar for the Florida Academy of Osteopathy. The other two lecturers were osteopaths Dick MacDonald and Herb Miller. I recall telling Dick that life felt like doing 30 days in jail—it was boring, I knew it would be over soon and I wished it would hurry up. Dick became a little angry with my dissatisfaction. He believed I had a lot of work to do yet while I thought I had done it all.

After the seminar was over, Dick offered to give me a treatment. I sat on the treatment table. In a very short time the top of my head was on the floor and my buttocks were still on the table. I was slightly hyperextended, to say the least, but it felt right. I was feeling releases that I never dreamed could happen. Pains and dysfunction that I had carried with me for a lot of years were popping loose.

Then we went into the recall of a very specific injury: I was an eleventh grader. It was the first football game of the season. I was the starting linebacker. On our first defensive play a hole opened on my side of the line and a huge farmer fullback was coming through. I put my head down and charged him like a bull. I remember a big noise when my helmet hit his thigh pad. I came back to conscious awareness in the fourth quarter of the game, over an hour later. I had often wondered why I'd been out of it so long. I was able to walk and talk but I didn't know what day it was or how many fingers the coach was holding up. I had total amnesia from the time of the tackle until I asked my friend Richard where I was.

During the treatment with Dick, I completely relived the experience. I hit the ball carrier's right thigh pad with the front of my helmet. My head snapped back and almost broke my neck. I could feel my head rotate slightly to the left. I felt, play by play, my head hyperextend on my atlas, then the cervical vertebra hyperextended one by one from upper to lower and then the upper thoracics hyperextended one by one down to the fifth. Next, the thoracolumbar junction and the right sacroiliac were mightily strained. I also felt a very sharp, sickening pain in the left knee. I had not remembered any of this before.

After the treatment I had a lot of aches and pains for a few days but it all felt right. During my recall of the collision with the ball carrier I felt a lot of energy go into my head. By the end of the treatment this energy was radiating out of my right forehead; this radiation continued for the rest of that day and about halfway through the next. I began to feel softer, less critical. My wife and children were astonished at the personality change I exhibited when I returned home from the seminar. I was tolerant of mistakes and errors. I was less arrogant and far more reasonable.

The experience raised several questions:

1. Can a head injury result in the long-term retention of an Energy Cyst?

2. Can that Energy Cyst result in personality changes?

3. Does release of an Energy Cyst result in reversal of the personality changes?

4. Could the same release be accomplished by CO_2 - O_2 therapy or psycho-therapy as well as by SomatoEmotional Release?

ACCEPTING TRAUMA FOR ANOTHER

I was about 4 years old and was playing out in front of our home on Cadillac Avenue in Detroit, Michigan. The four-lane street was rather busy, even in those days. There was a little girl who was probably 6 or 7 years old living across the street. We used to shout at each other across the street in an attempt to be friends. Neither of us was allowed to cross the street. The year was 1936.

It so happened that one summer day in late morning neither her parents nor mine were in view and we were both out in front of our respective houses shouting across the street to each other. As we conversed, we moved closer and closer to the street to hear each other better. Finally, it was decided that one of us should cross the street so that we could play together—since she was the older of the two of us, she would come over to my side of the street. She ran across the street between cars. She wasn't in my yard very long before she became frightened that her mother would discover she had broken the rules by coming over to see me.

I remember very vividly that she sort of panicked and ran into the street to get back to her side. When she was on the far side of the street she was hit by a car. I remember it clearly: The car hit her just above the right knee. She flew up in the air, landed on the car's fender and then fell off into the street. The noise of a horn and screeching brakes brought mothers out of the houses all up and down the street. The girl had fallen on the far side of the car. I couldn't see her. A man picked her up and carried her into another car and they drove away. I never saw her again.

The police came and there was a lot of confusion. I felt terribly guilty that she had come over to see me and been hit by a car. The police asked me (of all people) how fast the car was going when it hit the girl. I said, "Thirty-five miles per hour," because I'd heard my father mention that speed once while he was driving us somewhere. I really had no idea how fast the car was going. I hoped I hadn't gotten the car in trouble. The man who was driving the car that had hit her was crying.

In 1983, Dick MacDonald and I were trading treatments. He began my treatments with me standing. I felt pain in the lateral aspect of my right knee. Then my knee buckled medially. I went sideways onto the table then over the other side. Nothing like this had ever happened to me, but it felt very real and the releases were very powerful. Suddenly I completely recalled the incident I described above. I let go of a lot of energy, pain, fear and guilt. I let go of some more responsibility that day, too.

Now what? It would seem that it is possible to absorb an injury inflicted upon another person to whom you may be connected—emotionally, spiritually, by circumstance or who knows what. Perhaps I took on the girl's injury because I felt it was my fault that she was hit by a car. Since I never saw her again, I am very suspicious that she was killed.

ONCE AGAIN THE PROCESS DISPLAYS PERFECTION

During the last hour or two of the last afternoon of an Advanced Class in CranioSacral Therapy it has become my habit to give my body to the 10-person group for evaluation and treatment. (This is a seminar during which a lot of personal growth occurs for 99.9 percent of the participants. There have been a few holdouts, but very few. Forgive me, I digress. It is my purpose here to describe my experience as the patient for this specific group of excellent therapists, all of whom had demonstrated a remarkable degree of personal growth during the week.) A chief therapist is selected by the group.

In January 1988 as I lay on the table I experienced a sense of complete trust as Susan, the elected chief therapist, directed the placement of the other nine pairs of hands upon my body. I made little or no conscious attempt to analyze the process. It was very natural and easy to give myself over to it. In just a few minutes I began to vaguely move in and out of a sensation of birth. The sensation slowly solidified and I could feel the hands of William Naggs, M.D., on my head assisting the delivery process. My neck retracted. The therapist holding my head commented on the phenomenon. For just an instant I felt like a turtle pulling back into my shell. Then I seemed to be using my shoulders and arms against the inner rim of the birth canal to resist the doctor's pulling. Dr. Naggs was trying to help. I didn't see it that way.

Susan asked me something about why I didn't want to be born. That was not the issue. I became aware that the doctor was working against the natural delivery process—with good but misguided intention. I wanted to go slower so the process would be in keeping with nature's plan.

I shared this with Susan (I believe it was her) and she very wisely suggested that I tell the doctor to stop pulling and let nature take its course. I did and he honored my request. (After all, this was my fantasy.) For an unknown amount of time, I think quite a long while, I experienced the most remarkable and pleasant twisting and untwisting, relaxing and lengthening of my neck, torso and finally my legs. It felt like my first and to date most pleasant spinal manipulation treatment—no offense meant to those wonderful people who have applied their therapeutic skills to my body. (I now fully support Dick MacDonald's statement that the natural delivery process is the first spinal treatment. It is also the initiation to CranioSacral Therapy.) The process went slowly, unhurried by the doctor's pullings and urgings. I'm sure my reality changed by my request. My body lengthened and unwound beautifully. It gave me a beautiful experience as I left the safety of the womb to enter the outside world. A most remarkable sensation was the realization that one of the therapists (Scott) had a fist under my thorax at about T3 or T4. He seemed to be pushing inferiorly quite hard. This felt like my mother's pubes. Once I got past the pubes there were no further problems to overcome.

Then, one of the assistant therapists (Scott, I believe) asked if I'd had any problems with my heart or breathing at my delivery. I knew of none and I did not feel as though there were any at that time. Then it felt like about four hands and a forearm firmly pressing posteriorly onto/into the front of my thoracic cage. I then saw an image of my father. He was sad and tearful. He was at the delivery of his son. I suddenly realized my birth reminded him of the wife he'd had before my mother. This previous wife had borne him two daughters and then died of cancer. He married my mother. They conceived me and I was born on February 10, 1932. He was very sad. He still loved his deceased wife very much. I felt so much compassion for him that I accepted his grief into my body (lungs, the organs of grief in Chinese medicine) in order to help him. As I imagined this, he visibly brightened in countenance and his stature/posture straightened. I realized that I would take his grief and deal with it later in my own life—a lot of reasoning for a newborn, but it was very clear to me.

Then, a most remarkable realization occurred as the therapists helped me release the lung-based grief from my chest. I realized/knew that I had been meant to be born to my father and his first wife. Her death by cancer was not anticipated. Since we had contracted that he would be my father to begin this life, he had to find another mother for me. My mother never quite fit into the arrangement for as long as I remember. Now I know why; she was a second choice. Father loved her very much, but it just wasn't quite the same. What an insight this was for me.

Slowly, I returned to awareness of the here and now. I was amazed to realize that an hour and 45 minutes had passed. It was a beautiful experience. I felt wonderful and still do. It's really difficult to question the therapeutic process when experiences like this one are released from our memory banks. What a wonderful lesson. Thanks so much.

ANOTHER BREAKTHROUGH

The next Advanced Class treatment opened more doors than ever before. After placement of hands by the assistants, the chief therapist (Stan) began to gently but persistently push me into imagery and dialogue. I saw a black background with purple areas quite consistently. I had thoughts about accepting my father's grief as I described in the previous section. My left brain would not be quiet. I thought about many past experiences with SomatoEmotional Release work. Stan persisted.

I saw Dad's neon sign on the porch at 5706 Cadillac Avenue. The sign said Notary Public. He was teaching me to read it inside out. It was night. I was on the front porch swing. Dad didn't have to serve eviction notices anymore. Mom wanted me in bed. If I kept looking at the red neon sign I didn't have to go to bed. I saw a black border with a purple center again. A shiny spot developed in the purple center. The spot was like a purple-violet radiant crystal. With some urging from Stan, the crystal came closer and became larger. It turned silver. I kept looking at the silver area. Then I saw a face in it that looked like a porpoise face.

Without hesitation Stan asked me the "porpoise" (purpose) of that face. I was amused and relaxed by his play on words. The humor he injected seemed to ease the barrier with which I was struggling. The porpoise face turned into a spaceship. The spaceship had a voice. It began to communicate, first with me and then with the rest of the group through me. The points of discussion—which I remember so well—were:

1.   The occupants weren't quite sure whether I was ready to receive what they were going to communicate to me.

2.   I was one of them but I had been assigned to earth for about five thousand years and had experienced many lifetimes during this five thousand year assignment. I should not get caught up in the earthly life, however. I must always know that I am an envoy from beyond.

3.   My assignment from the beginning of my time on earth has been to "soften" the earth's inhabitants. One of the ways we are doing this is by the teaching of "soft touch." CranioSacral Therapy and ShareCare are presented in order to teach soft touch and thus allay fear and reduce anger and frustration. Soft touch promotes love and union.

4.   We come from infinity far beyond any present-day conceptual scientific framework on earth.

5.   The God of earthlings is a subsidiary of the God of the Universe. Earthlings' concepts of the universe are diminutive compared to what is really out there.

6.   Our planet is like a person. It is our mother. The softening of earth people through soft touch and love will cause the Mother Earth to be loved and respected by those she supports. She deserves love and respect. She gives so unselfishly and without question. Her gifts are running out.

My mother gave me toughness, my father gave me compassion this time. Both are necessary for this task.

When I was asked by the chief therapist if there were others present from the same place, I pointed—with my eyes closed—around one of the therapists to a table on the other side of the room where Stan's wife (they tell me) had just come in and laid down.

Time will tell. I don't know what this experience means but it was sobering and wondrous.

MORE FROM THE ADVANCED CLASS

Three months later, almost as soon as the 10 pairs of hands were upon me in a gentle, energy-providing way, I began to see images. First I saw and felt as though I were in a cylinder made of Lucite or some other transparent material. I was very calm and felt as though everything was going as it was supposed to. Then I was ejected from the cylinder as though from a torpedo tube. I headed through space toward planet Earth. I circled a few times and came down some distance from a castle fortress. This building was teeming with barbarians. There was a moat with a drawbridge.

I was off in a distance in some trees and they had not seen me. I looked down at myself and realized I was in the wrong uniform. I wanted to go into the fortress, blend in and be inconspicuous. I had on a rather snappy-looking Nazi officer-type uniform. I found I had the ability to change my uniform by thought, and I changed it to the raggedy-looking type of clothing the soldiers were wearing. I needed to get closer to make myself and my garb more appropriate, but I couldn't see the details from this distance. I began to walk closer. I got very close. Then my concern over the proper attire and demeanor faded away because I realized the barbarian-type soldiers couldn't see me. I was invisible. I entered the castle fortress and looked around at the soldiers milling about. Many were chewing meat off bones. They were talking loudly and sometimes waving the bones at each other. "Hussars" was the name that came to mind when the therapists asked who these people were.

We were in the Eastern European part of the world. It was late afternoon. It was rather cold. Snow patches were here and there. Upon looking around, I realized that this was not going to be a good place for me to do my work, so I left. It was beautiful. I was invisible so I just flew away. I notified my home base that I was changing locations. I seemed to soar effortlessly around the Earth a few times, then I saw a sign that read "Tennessee" on a white background in the shape of that state. It was on a continent that looked like North America.

I went to Tennessee. As I approached, the map-like image turned into the state's proper topography. I landed on a battlefield. I became a Tennessee Volunteer soldier. I had a bandage wrapped around my left shoulder axilla and upper thorax. There was a lot of blood. I knew that I had a musket ball in my axilla pressing against my upper ribs and shoulder joint. I elected to keep this situation. A Yankee Civil War surgeon was preparing to remove the musket ball from my body. He had a cautery iron in the fire which would be used to heat sterilize the wound after he took the musket ball out of my armpit. I felt detached. I knew if I were to gather information about the strange fascination that Earth inhabitants seem to have with pain, I would have to experience this pain and see what was so enjoyable about it.

As the musket ball was being removed in my imagery, the therapists were delivering a large Energy Cyst from my left armpit. The synchronization of the two events was perfect. Then the imaged surgeon sterilized my wound with the red hot cautery iron. I got no joy from any of this. I remained puzzled about why Earth people continue to do these things to each other.

I reported my experience and my impressions to my home base and returned to an outpost for repairs and rejuvenation. The mission was a failure. I was trying to discover why Earth people continue to inflict and suffer pain, destruction and death. Reason told me that there must be some joy involved in it. But as I experienced the pain of the musket ball removal and heat cautery, my earthly body felt no joy or satisfaction. I still don't understand.

A QUIET ONE

I received my next Advanced Class treatment in September 1988—a very quiet, rejuvenating experience. During the five-day class, one of the students (Toni) presented a guide for her treatments named "Ramus." He became so prominent during the class that the group elected him chief therapist and, thus, in charge of my treatment.

Ramus instructed the class to put healing, no-strings-attached generic energy into my body. As this went on, I felt Ramus was scanning my skeletal structure for chips, dents and weak spots and repairing them. Then he went through my muscles, ligaments and tendons, repairing each damaged area as he went. (He did not do anything with my viscera. It was not said but I sensed that visceral healing was not appropriate at that time.) It was a wonderful, quiet, non-sensational experience. I felt serene when it was over, as if I had been oiled, greased, overhauled and tuned up.

PIECE OF INSIGHT, NOVEMBER 1988

The next Advanced Class in November 1988 gave me a very nice recharging treatment. My chief therapist (Chris) asked my Inner Physician to please come forward. A huge, wonderful, kind, gentle and absolutely non-threatening gorilla appeared.

He said that I should not forget that I was one of his descendants. He told me I had wondered for some time what purpose the herds of grazing animals such as the wildebeest, reindeer and caribou serve on this planet. They eat grass and fertilize to grow more grass, but what does all this contribute to the ecosystem? He explained that all grazing herds are producers of positive thought forms. Their product is necessary to counterbalance the negative thought forms produced by so many humans and some other animals. That was our lesson for the day.

MORE FUN

The Advanced Class in May 1989 treated me very well. Shari was the chief therapist. I had two guides present themselves during my session. Reynaldo and Umberto were their names.

Reynaldo was very serious. He let me know that I had much work to do. This work all related to the study of the motivation behind violence and the destructive activities in which so many earth people indulge. He told me that the work done so far was good, but if the earth was to be salvaged there was not much time to waste.

Umberto, on the other hand, was insistent that we all have some fun. We need to dance and drink wine. He said that he and I and Shari had lived together in Florence. We were all lovers and partners. We shared a wonderful life at that time.

This seemed to be a lesson in balance between serious work and real fun.

CONFIRMATION

The July 1989 Advanced Class experience was one of confirmation and expansion. I recited to the class words that came from somewhere—but which I had not considered before. I'm not sure where they came from.

My chief therapist (Lisa) went a little fast in the beginning. She said she had never treated a no-resistance patient before. As I offered no resistance, she didn't know quite what to do, so she talked. Once past that, I began to recite.

In essence, I said the following:

1. There are specific nuclei in the human brain which are activated by violent, destructive and homicidal behavior. It is a similar phenomenon to the thrill seeker activity that many people pursue. When activated, these nuclei give a sense of pleasure and gratification.

2. CranioSacral Therapy stimulates the development of brain nuclei that balance the effect of these violence-responding nuclei. There is more to CranioSacral Therapy than touch and structure: The energy input positively affects chromosomal development and control. It stimulates the development of these "loving behavior" nuclei.

3. The pleasure produced by violent, destructive and homicidal behavior is tempered and modulated by CranioSacral Therapy. Further, these newly-developing balance nuclei give pleasure from loving activity.

4. It all fits together with an evolving chromosomal modification that is in process.

5. If the negative energy level becomes high enough, the surface of the earth could and would spontaneously incinerate. Although we are not near that level at present, we must not become complacent.

The process is working and the level of joy derived from violent and destructive behavior is topping off. We must continue the work.

CLOSING

In this chapter, I have shared with you some very personal experiences that have made an impact on my life and development. I'm not trying to convince you of anything, just reporting my experiences. You can make of them what you wish. I do hope this sharing will help open your mind as these experiences have opened mine.

Once the mind is open, it would seem that things begin to happen that cause further opening. It is as though the powers that be see a chink in our armor and know we are thereafter more and more amenable to further opening.

I'm not in possession of the meaning of my reported experiences. I am comfortable with the realization that there is a tremendous amount of stuff out there that I don't know about. I hope to increase your comfort level with this same realization.

Chapter VII
Channeling ???

*Whether it's true or imaginary, I have learned from the experience
and am thankful.*

John E. Upledger, D.O., O.M.M.

As you continue to work with such characterizations as Inner Physicians, Higher Consciousness and Inner Wisdom, there is an excellent chance you will encounter a situation that sounds and feels like you are in communication with an entity outside the patient's immediate and personal consciousness. Some call it "channeling." That is, you may feel that you are speaking with a disincarnate guide who is involved with the patient on an esoteric or spiritual level. If you need to know whether this is true, you have a real problem because to prove or disprove such a situation is well nigh impossible.

Arguments can be made that the "spirit guide" is a figment of the patient's imagination. Similarly, any clinical changes that might occur after conversations and encounters between therapeutic facilitators and spirit guides might well happen secondary to suggestion, therapeutic imagery, placebo and the like. On the other hand, phenomena sometimes occur that make it so difficult to explain what you have witnessed in non-spiritual terms that it seems more rational to entertain a spiritual guide explanation rather than continue to stretch logic to remain skeptical and continue in a more traditional or scientific frame of mind.

In the final analysis, it is up to each individual patient and therapeutic facilitator team to determine whether they believe there has been contact and assistance or resistance from a spiritual entity or not. I believe it matters little what the personal belief system of the therapeutic facilitator allows. When working with a patient, I suggest the practitioner make it a rule to not disagree with any belief system or circumstance the patient presents, so long as it rings true and is verified with the craniosacral rhythm (when it is used as a Significance Detector). You should blend with patients, becoming part of them. Leave personal beliefs and prejudices outside the treatment room door.

I know that I can't cop out on the questions about channeling that easily, but suspension of my belief system is my personal code of therapeutic facilitator conduct. As for my beliefs, I think it is best to describe some experiences that have influenced my present feelings about such matters. Then, you may better understand the "how and why" of my belief system. I have described some of my experiences as a participant in Chapter VI. The experiences I am about to recount all occurred while I was in the therapeutic facilitator role.

I have worked for several years with patients' nonconscious. Frequently, the nonconscious seems quite distant from the central focus of conscious awareness.

The nonconscious often seems shy and withdrawn. It may require a great deal of gentle, patient urging to bring it to the foreground where it will begin communication with both the patient's conscious and you.

The First Encounter:
Frederick, Doctor of Internal Medicine Calls in a Consultant

It was in one of those situations of deep relaxation coupled with intense concentration that my first experience of possible communication with a patient's disincarnate spiritual guide occurred. Since that first experience this type of phenomenon has often reoccurred.

The first time was in 1984. This patient was a very pleasant practicing psychologist/psychotherapist. She was middle-aged and in chronic left arm, shoulder, upper thoracic, cervical and head pain since an automobile accident two years earlier. She had been through the therapeutic spectrum with orthopedics, physical therapy, chiropractic and biofeedback. I did not find a structural basis for her pain but there seemed to be excessive retention of multiple, traumatically induced Energy Cysts.

As we were working with the Energy Cyst release process, combined with some SomatoEmotional Release of materials that predated the automobile accident, I enlisted the aid of her Inner Physician who came forward in a very helpful and accommodating manner. The Inner Physician was named Frederick. He was most cooperative as he confirmed when the precise body positions for Energy Cyst releases were achieved. He told us when the maximum release had been exploited from a given position.

He informed us that a lot of retention of the traumatic energy from the automobile accident was due to retained resentment and smoldering anger resultant to the dissolution of the patient's 22-year marriage that had ended in 1978. There were five grown children from this marriage.

As I worked with the patient and Frederick over a half-dozen sessions, my relationship with Frederick became more and more cordial and relaxed. (The patient was totally unaware of our conversations.) Frederick let me know that the end of the pain syndrome would not occur until the ill feelings of the marriage had been completely resolved. I continued to ask Frederick how we could best achieve this final release of resentment and anger. Frederick gave some advice, but he seemed a little vague and unsure of himself as we continued to attempt to gain acceptance and resolution of the divorce. Our efforts in this direction were not totally successful.

During the sixth session, I asked Frederick if there might be a consultant available who he could invite into our conversations—one who might be willing and able to advise us regarding the last residuum of the pain syndrome and the related resentment and anger. As a rather experienced psychologist/psychotherapist, this patient was not easily moved toward total resolution of the ill will she continued to

harbor against her ex-husband. She had her defenses well in place. She had toler-
ated several episodes of his unfaithfulness and philandering; the thanks she got for
her tolerance (which is often enabling behavior in disguise) was that her husband
finally asked for a divorce. This really hurt her pride and gave her a chance to
develop an unhealthy level of self-righteous anger and a lust for revenge.

When we asked for a consultant to come forward, the patient's voice became
very deep and developed an accent I could not identify. It was a little difficult to
understand. The new voice announced his name was EUPHEMUS.[21] He spelled it
for me. He was not of her nonconscious (I used the word "subconscious" at that
time), rather he had been "assigned" to help her deal with a problem plaguing her
for several hundred years. EUPHEMUS further explained that he had guided her
to me because he knew I was "open" and would allow him and others to work
through me.

I decided to go along with the scenario. I asked EUPHEMUS whether we had
known each other before. He exclaimed, "Certainly! How could you have forgotten our time together, both in Ancient Greece and in Egypt?" I kept my wits about
me and reminded the slightly insulted EUPHEMUS that I was Earthbound at
present. According to the way things work here on Earth, I had amnesia for my
previous spiritual existences and in large part for my previous Earth incarnations.
EUPHEMUS apologized for having forgotten how things worked for you when
you are incarnate on earth. He would keep this in mind and be patient with me. In
any case, EUPHEMUS said that we had been healers together in Egypt. Before
that, he had known of me in Greece where I was a rather precocious and rebellious
young healer in training. He told me that I was well-known throughout the Medi-
terranean world during the fourth century B.C. In fact, I was too well-known. I
demonstrated my talents without discretion. Thus, I was beheaded at the age of 12
by politically oriented and envious teachers. EUPHEMUS told me that three of
the principal teachers who were responsible for my death were on Earth right now,
and they would like to repeat my decapitation. He told me that I was not in any
great danger now but that I should beware of jealousy and exercise caution. I thanked
EUPHEMUS for the advice. I assured him I would be alert for danger and changed
the subject back to the patient.

According to EUPHEMUS, this patient had been in Atlantis. He stated that
during that incarnation she had been responsible in part for her present day ex-
husband's loss of reputation, his ultimate demise and the attendant shame with
which he died. EUPHEMUS explained that the patient must recognize that the
disagreement and vengeful attitude between them had been going on over several
Earth lifetime interrelationships. The problems would continue until both of them

---

[21] Throughout this section, the names of spirit guides are indicated via all upper case letters to differentiate them from the
names of Inner Physicians, Inner Wisdom, Tumors.

were willing to accept equal responsibility for their ongoing problems and to forget vengeance. It would go on until this patient accepted the fact that what her ex-husband had done was unimportant in the grand scheme of things. Then and only then would there be no further need for the pain that had brought her to see me.

I asked EUPHEMUS how I might promote resolution between these two souls. He instructed me to gradually enlighten this patient to tolerance about the reasons for her symptoms. He warned me to not tell her too much all at once. I broached the subject after she returned to conscious awareness. The patient was very receptive and seemed willing to work on resolution of a problem that began several centuries before in Atlantis. I had three more sessions with the patient after this initial conversation with EUPHEMUS. She got complete relief of pain.

EUPHEMUS encouraged me to continue to be open. He also told me "they" would be using my services a lot more now that I was open. He bade me good-bye for awhile and told me not to worry. I was doing as they would like me to do. He also told me that he thought this patient could resolve the rest of her problem with their help. He did not anticipate that she would require any more of my services, but if another obstacle proved difficult, he would see to it that she would return to me. About six months later she returned for two mundane visits during which I mostly did energy work with her liver and the second and fourth chakra energy centers. There was no contact with EUPHEMUS. She is doing fine now.

I really did not know what to make of this experience so I did not reject or accept it as literally true. I could make a case for the psychology of forgiveness with pride and dignity painting such a scenario, but I felt as though I would be reaching to stay on familiar ground. So I decided not to decide but rather to remain open and see what might happen next.

Theo and the Actress

Four days after my final communication with EUPHEMUS, an actress in her mid-sixties came in as a patient. Her complaints were of syncope and dizziness. She had suffered these symptoms for some 15 years. Of late, the symptoms had become worse so that they interfered with her ability to perform. She feared she might stagger or faint while on stage. It hadn't happened yet, but the attendant apprehension interfered with her confidence and, thus, her ability to give herself up to her part. She also had a clearly structural somatic dysfunction of the sixth rib on the right side that she stated interfered with her ability to breathe deeply.

She was seated on the treatment table and I was behind her with my hands on the posterior rib cage to evaluate rib function. This was during the first few minutes of our visit. She seemed to go into a trance as I had my hands on her posterior ribs. Almost immediately a deep voice came from her. The voice said, "Don't worry about the ribs, my son. That problem will be very easy to correct—or it may correct itself once she has accepted herself into her present reality." Astonished, I wrote this quote down so I wouldn't forget. My mind jumped from astonished to skeptical. I began to make up reasons for her conduct that related to her being a melodramatic actress, perhaps having multiple personality disorder, being totally crazy and so on.

Then the voice told me she had been directed to me because I was open. I translated this as a suggestion that I suspend my skepticism and open myself to what was happening. I was successful at getting my own baggage out of the room. The voice went on and told both of us—for she was able to remember everything after the session—that there were several souls who wanted to communicate with her but that she was afraid. Because of this fear, she had been rejecting communication for a long time. I asked the deep voice by what name I could address it. The name given was "THEO."

I asked THEO if we had met before. He said, "No," but he had heard of my healing abilities when I was an apprentice in ancient Greece. He told me that I was well-known and created much jealousy in my elders because of my popularity. He then told me to be careful because they had beheaded me once while I was quite young. I shouldn't let it happen again. He also told me that because I was open, I would be used frequently to help souls who were having difficulties getting past certain obstacles. They could put what I needed to know into my head and I would be able to help these souls get back on the path.

I saw this woman three times at monthly intervals. I had no more contact with THEO, but she seemed to communicate a great deal with her grandfather who had died about 20 years earlier. There seemed to be a lot of advice passed from him to her. As she was able to accept her grandfather's presence without fear, the syncope and dizzy spells ended, as did her fear of their occurrence. (The rib problem was easily corrected at the end of the first session using direct thrust.) I have not seen this patient since the end of that third session. Singularly, this experience with THEO would have been easy to dismiss were it not coupled with the previously described experience regarding the story of my decapitation in Greece. It was a little more difficult not to accept the experiences at face value.

Next came the clincher.

Bob, Gordon and CAUTHUS

About a week after my encounter with THEO, a 42-year-old male named Bob came from the Northeast for a week of treatments. This meant that I would work with him through regular 45-minute sessions on Monday, Tuesday, Thursday and Friday of that week.

Monday was a quiet visit; I did most of the steps of the 10-step protocol easily. Tuesday I completed the mouth and TMJ work. I was not yet deeply into the hyoid and throat work. Toward the end of the session, I asked why he had come to see me; there didn't seem to be any major areas of dysfunction or pain. Bob said he just wanted to experience the work for which I was rather well known. He said he could afford the luxury.

Thursday, he started a SomatoEmotional Release that involved an old back injury that had occurred while he was a teenage hockey player. He had fallen on the ice. He was mortified. He felt himself a fool. No one had pushed or checked him. He was not scrambling for the puck. He was skating up the ice in relative peace when his feet went faster than the rest of his body. It was a Sunday. He was playing hockey for a local dry cleaners' team. His father was watching. He was really embarrassed and angry with himself. We re-experienced the fall on his coccyx. We released an Energy Cyst from his low lumbar area via the coccygeal route. Along with the Energy Cyst came the release of embarrassment, mortification and some self-abuse. He really cussed himself out. He apologized to his father who was very understanding. He finally saw the humor of the whole situation and laughed at himself.

By this time, he was in a deep, pleasant state of relaxation. I asked his Inner Physician if we could talk. The Inner Physician said, "Of course." His Inner Physician's name was "Gordon." Gordon said that what we had done would help Bob's self-esteem significantly and that there was nothing else to do that day, but the next day we had a special project to complete.

Friday, Bob arrived for his last in the series of four appointments. He was to fly home that evening. Bob said that he'd had a good night. He also said that he had gotten in touch with a lot of self-criticism to which he had been subjecting himself. He thought that was over now. He really had a much nicer feeling about himself and his abilities. I didn't think he would have to go on proving himself so much from now on.

I began the session with a CV-4. Bob went into a state of deep relaxation almost immediately. I asked Gordon if he would care to join us. Gordon responded that he was already present and that he wanted to introduce someone to me. I indicated I would be most honored to meet anyone Gordon wanted to introduce. Gordon introduced me to CAUTHUS.

CAUTHUS' voice was different, a softer yet more firm voice. CAUTHUS said, "It is a pleasure to meet you, my son." He told me that it was he who had directed Bob to see me and that he was satisfied with what had been accomplished. I indicated that I was surprised that one so evolved as CAUTHUS should be interested in the resolution of the residue of a fall on the ice. CAUTHUS became just a little impatient. He let me know that the work we accomplished was much deeper than the fall. He also let me know that he was surprised that I was not aware of that. I told CAUTHUS that I simply followed my hands and let whatever happens happen. I tried not to get in the way. CAUTHUS' voice softened again and he said, "Of course, my son. You are open. That is why we can work through you."

I then followed my impulse and asked CAUTHUS if we had known each other before. CAUTHUS told me that he had hoped to study healing with me in ancient Greece but that I had been slain by a politicized group of healers before he had the chance. I almost fell off my stool! This was the third time I had been told this same story by the spiritual guides of three different patients who, at least in the here and now, did not know each other. CAUTHUS told me that when you are working out on the edge, there will always be those who try to strike you down.

Three times in three weeks I was told by seemingly independent sources that I had been terminated in ancient Greece by physicians or would-be healers because I was overly precocious and gaining a reputation. All three gave gentle warnings about present-day professional jealousies. All three said that they had directed these patients to me because I was "open." It becomes very difficult to discount the authenticity of the information when it comes at you from three separate directions at the same time.

Yes, I do believe that spirit guides are real. And I know deep inside of me that if you will go with the flow of things, these guides will tell you precisely what should be done and how to direct your life. It is since the experiences recounted above that I have arrived at the knowledge that spirit guides are real. This is not rational belief; it is gut level knowledge. Now that I am "open," I have had several experiences with patients wherein these guides have played key roles.

Samantha and Her Group of International Guides

At this point, I should like to present a most remarkable clinical case which was more deeply involved with spirit guides than I could have ever imagined. I could easily see why I may have had so many preliminary experiences simply in preparation for this very complex and very needy 37-year-old lady. I will call her "Samantha" in order to protect her privacy. She is not, however, overly concerned with privacy. She has recounted her experiences to one SomatoEmotional Release class and three Advanced CranioSacral Therapy classes.

Samantha was a successful business executive at the time of her first visit on February 4, 1988. She had been on the fast track as a business professional for about 15 years prior to this meeting. She had suffered from endometriosis during her early twenties. This is a condition that creates painful menstrual cycles because uterine lining tissue is located in places outside the uterus. When a menstrual cycle occurs, there is bleeding from this abnormally located uterine lining tissue. Blood cysts may be formed in the lining of the pelvic cavity, on the bowel, on the outside of the uterus, ovaries, tubes, ligaments, etc. It can be quite a painful condition. She stated that she had been successfully treated with some kind of medication but could not remember what it was. She had been on birth control pills on and off for about 10 years. She had discontinued their use about two years prior to this visit. She had not been married, nor had she been pregnant. She smoked 20 to 30 filter cigarettes per day and had done so for several years. She claimed only moderate use of alcohol. She had been sexually active, in moderation, for several years.

The reason for this visit—and it was an emergency visit that was filled into a cancellation appointment—was that about three months earlier she had discovered a suspicious lump in her left breast during a self-examination. Two days prior to this visit, she had undergone an evaluation by another physician. She had undergone a mammogram, Sonogram and Trans Illumination evaluation of the breasts. She had previously had a mammogram and breast evaluation in November 1986 at which time only fibrocystic breast disease was noted.

At this time, all three tests showed a suspicious mass in the left breast of about 2 centimeters by 0.5 centimeters in size. This mass was attached to a smaller round mass about 1.1 centimeters in diameter. No masses were noted in the axillae. The right breast showed no suspicious masses, but both breasts had dense fibrocystic tissue with a small proportion of fat.

My own manual examination at this time was done without knowledge of the above test results. I reviewed the reports after I had done my own examination. I recorded the presence of a suspicious mass at 11 o'clock in the left breast, just above the nipple. The mass was attached to the deep side of the skin, which made it very suspicious for malignancy. I estimated its size at about 3 centimeters by 1.5 centimeters with an almost vertical longitudinal axis in an almost vertical direction. I could find no suspicious masses in either of the axillae. Both breasts presented the tissue texture of typical fibrocystic disease.

After my examination, our discussion of my findings and the implications thereof, I asked Samantha why she had come to see me with such an urgent problem. She said that she had heard of alternative methods of treatment for breast cancer and that she would like to know more about them and perhaps give them a try. I suggested that the alternative methods might be a little slow at this stage of the game and that they might better be integrated with the surgeon's work and used as an adjunct. She then told me that she was scheduled for a mastectomy on February 19, 1988. That gave us two weeks to see what we might be able to do.

I explained the concepts of Therapeutic Imagery and Dialogue to her. She seemed receptive and eager to try this approach. During the CV-4, she became very relaxed. She was able to visualize a quiet beach on which she and I were sunning ourselves. (I wanted to be included in her images right from the start.) We then invited her Inner Physician to join us.

Her Inner Physician seemed eager to accept our invitation. His name was Harold. He told us the tumor in her breast was malignant and its name was Black Mass. Harold suggested that "White Love" in the heart could hold the tumor in abeyance. He clearly understood that "Black Mass" could and would kill Samantha.

Black Mass then spoke to us. He stated that he was tired of living with anger and without love. He would prefer that Samantha die and begin over again with a better attitude. This was a very powerful stance to take at an initial meeting. I negotiated with Black Mass and Samantha. I asked that since the situation was very urgent, could we please shrink the tumor temporarily and use pain to maintain Samantha's attention and keep her aware of the power of Black Mass. That was agreeable to Black Mass. Harold thought it was a good idea and suggested that the pain should be in the toes of the right foot. Black Mass agreed. Then, Harold suggested that I put "loving energy" into Samantha's heart and concentrate, with intention to shrink the tumor. I did my best to follow Harold's suggestions. After about five minutes of concentrated intention, there was a palpable "snap" in the tumor area after about five minutes of concentrated intention. By the time we were finished with the first session, the palpable size of the tumor was reduced by about 50 percent.

When Samantha came back to the here and now, she had no conscious memory of the events that had occurred. She did not remember Harold or Black Mass. I described the session to her and had her feel her tumor. She was astonished to note that there was a significant reduction in the tumor's size and hardness from just an hour before. She was reinforced to the extent that I felt quite optimistic about what we would be able to do with this problem.

I asked her about anger and love. She mentioned sexual molestation as a child by both her father and a man named George. We didn't have time to pursue it at that time. She said she thought she had dealt with these problems previously. It didn't seem important to me either. Neither of us felt we could afford to be diverted from focusing on the tumor at that time since surgery was imminent.

Samantha's next visit was eight days later, on February 12, 1988. This was one week before her surgery. The tumor in the left breast was still about one-half the size it had been at the beginning of the first visit. I must confess, I was probably as excited about this as Samantha.

As I put my hands on her head to begin the session, Samantha went right off into an altered state of consciousness. I asked Harold, her Inner Physician, to join us. Harold said he had been helping to clear residual anger and that things were looking pretty good.

Then a voice from Samantha spoke with a very powerful British accent. I really had no idea where this voice came from. I asked who the voice was and it said, "John, have you forgotten me already?" I was totally astonished but tried to not show it. I tried to keep my cool. I explained to this voice that being incarnate and earthbound interfered with memories of past incarnations and spiritual existences. I asked who the voice was. He said his name was HAWKINS. He said that we had worked together in biological research at Cambridge about 200 years ago. He told me that I was always too serious and that he frequently had to take me out of the laboratory to relax. He always took me to a pub where we drank ale and "pinched bottoms."

HAWKINS said he was one of "those" who was assigned to Samantha. They knew I would work with them, so they had directed her to me. HAWKINS said she was redeemable and could do a lot of good work if she could be guided past certain obstacles. He was sure we could save her from the cancer.

HAWKINS then suggested that she visualize white blood cells digesting the cancer. He also directed me in putting energy directly through the breast. He said he would work with me. I could feel his presence. Then Harold suggested we release the Black Mass energy into space. We—rather I—could feel the release occur. At the end of the session, the tumor felt about the size of a pea. HAWKINS suggested that I teach Samantha to visualize the white blood cells digesting any cancer remnants. He thought she might not require surgery if we worked fast enough.

Samantha once again awakened with no recall of the session. She felt her lump and immediately realized that it was much smaller. I instructed her on the visualization technique of having the white blood cells (they looked like Pacman) digesting any tumor remnants that were there. She said she would do this visualization daily. When she asked me about her sore right fifth toe, I responded in a very noncommittal way. I pondered about this HAWKINS fellow.

On February 19, 1988, Samantha underwent what was described as a "breast biopsy" because the surgeon was struck with how much smaller the tumor was now. The mastectomy was not done as planned. The tissue that was removed was 1 centimeter in diameter. It contained mucinous carcinoma. The pathologist did not believe that the tumor was completely excised. There was confusion because the surgeon felt that the mass was totally removed. I can't help but wonder if the surgery had taken a time frame study of a malignant tumor in retrogression/regression rather than in an aggressive/invasive stage. It is seldom that I have seen this kind of confusion on reports. All of the other laboratory tests, x-rays, electrocardiographs and physical examinations were within the normal ranges and limits.

Samantha's next visit with me was on February 26, 1988, just one week after her breast surgery. She had recovered uneventfully from her surgery. She was excited because the surgeon was puzzled about the rapid regression in the size of the cancer. She was to go to the surgeon for a biopsy on the other breast just to be sure. This was the kind of cancer that often strikes both breasts. That biopsy was scheduled for February 28, 1988, just two days later. Samantha's faith in her own self-healing power was not yet strong enough to resist the second biopsy suggestion. She would follow the recommendations of the gynecologist for the right breast biopsy but she would not have the previously recommended left breast mastectomy with radiation and chemotherapy to follow.

As I put my hands on Samantha's head, she went into her altered consciousness almost immediately. My office assistant was with me now because things had been getting too complicated for me to remember it all. I would not be able to record it accurately and completely on the chart after my hands were free. We asked the Inner Physician to please consult with us. A Dr. Visor came on the scene. He told us that anticancer white blood cells were his specialty. They were manufactured in the bone marrow. Samantha said later, during our conversation at the end of the session, that she knew nothing about white blood cells and where they came from. Dr. Visor advised large doses of Vitamin B complex and Vitamin C from now on. He also said that Samantha should take three large glasses of carrot juice daily as well as supplemental zinc, calcium, chromium and selenium, all in the chelated form. She was also to take the enzymes bromelene and papase.

After this consultation with Dr. Visor, I was inspired to ask who was in charge of the cancer process anyway. This was when Big C came forward. A deep, ominous voice came forth from Samantha's very feminine vocal apparatus and told us he was in charge. He informed us that the cancer had come because of the male hormone Danocine which Samantha had been given for the endometriosis many years ago and because of a mineral deficiency. It was now Big C's purpose to draw Samantha's attention to her female side which had been partially subdued by the Danocine. He further stated that the minerals advised by Dr. Visor were necessary to restore femininity.

I negotiated with Big C. I told him that he had Samantha's attention and that I would see to it that she knew she would have to get feminine. Negotiation was difficult because Samantha was "out of it" and could not be brought into the conversation. It felt like we were negotiating her fate without her having any input. I felt like a lawyer must feel trying to avoid the death penalty for a client. In any case, Big C agreed to surrender some of his cancer cells. He gave some up to the white cells and he agreed that the molecular structure of some of the malignant cells were to be converted back to normal and that those malignant cells would then return to normal function and status. At this time, I was instructed to put energy in through the Crown Chakra. I was then told to invite Samantha to join us.

This time she responded, although still in a deep trance. She was told to visualize Big C putting on a white coat. (He had been wearing a black cape.) Samantha was successful in putting the white coat on Big C. I was then instructed to put energy through the left thorax and breast. When this was done, I was instructed to put energy into the right breast; Big C said he had two cancer cells in the right breast as an insurance policy.

Next, an Oriental-accented voice was heard. That voice belonged to an entity who introduced himself as LU CHOW PIN. He said he was helping with the energy. LU CHOW PIN was another of the guides assigned to this case along with HAWKINS. While I was getting acquainted with LU CHOW PIN, I simply followed my hands and released the throat, left arm and then the pubes, to help the hormones. LU CHOW PIN said, "You smart man, blessing all," and left the session. Big C felt good that Samantha would become a woman as her first priority.

He agreed to wear the white coat for a while. (I assumed this meant he would withhold further malignant activity.)

On February 28, 1988, Samantha went into the hospital for a biopsy of the right breast. No malignancy was found at that time. The biopsy report on the left breast was finalized; it was then officially called a colloid carcinoma of the left breast, less than 1 centimeter in diameter. (An official—if not real—end to the confusion of the first biopsy.) It appeared that Samantha had made significant progress toward the solution of her problem.

Samantha came to see me again on March 2, just one month after her first visit: a lot of water under the bridge for all of us in a short (February) month. At this session, we thought we would be smart and audio tape it from start to finish. We did. We listened to it once, and it was fine. We tried to listen again in another week and all we heard was static. I mention the audio tape self-destructing because I need the excuse for my sketchy notes on this session. I relied on the audio tape. Fortunately, I also had two preceptors with me who helped reconstruct the happenings.

This session was largely conducted by spirit guide LU CHOW PIN. Samantha spoke again with an Oriental accent with an inscrutable expression on her face. It was most remarkable. LU CHOW PIN recommended that Samantha drink tahebo tea and that she make poultices of tahebo bark to be placed over the ovaries and breasts for 30 minutes daily. He also advised Samantha to take ginseng. He said it was imperative that she restore her femininity which had been disturbed by early sexual molestation, by the Danocine (male hormone she took for her endometriosis) and by her yang existence in the male business world. LU CHOW PIN also told us that LURIE, a great master, was watching. He told us that Big C's attitude and his energy had further softened. He was still a little suspicious and defensive, but not bad. This was a great session. (I only wish that I had not relied on the audio tape, that my notes were more extensive.)

Samantha felt wonderful when it was over, but we had to instruct her about everything because she had no idea of what had happened. She accepted the instructions about tahebo tea, the poultices and the ginseng. By this time, she was getting used to strange instructions and strange explanations.

Samantha came for her next session on March 4. I only had to touch her head once she was in the supine position and she assumed the character of LU CHOW PIN immediately. LU CHOW PIN told me that the cancer was all gone. A new character named Luke was to keep the white blood cells active and in good number. Big C was happy. We just did routine hands-on work, got to know LU CHOW PIN better and had fun.

The next time Samantha visited was on March 31, about four weeks later. This time lapse told me she was trusting herself and the expertise and power of her protector spiritual guides. I chatted with both LU CHOW PIN and HAWKINS.

They both agreed that all was going well. Samantha would now be allowed some grace time to get it together so that she could become a true female. She also had to begin her assigned work which was to help others to evolve. She was not to continue working in the primitive monetary world of business. I could tell her this, but I was to be gentle and not scare her off. LU CHOW PIN added that the yin (left) side of her body was still confused. I should put energy through it to help it to organize. Also, if she didn't show progress toward the development of helping her feminine side, she would get pain on the left side. There would be no more cancer unless she rebelled against her new life.

I did not see Samantha again until September 15, 1988. She had gone to New York where her parents lived. While she was there, she was persuaded by family and friends—who thought it was an act of suicide to refuse mastectomy, radiation and chemotherapy—to undergo a complete medical workup. No one could find any signs of cancer. The fact that she had undergone a lot of criticism and intimidation was apparent, however. She had more self-doubt than she'd had the first time I had seen her. She was also complaining of left arm, shoulder and neck pain. She was afraid that this was a cancer recurrence.

During this session, Samantha went deeply into her usual trance. First EKETAN introduced himself. He stated that he personally had taken charge of Samantha's case because it was time for her to demonstrate the depth of her faith. He told me to spend as much time with her as seemed advisable because she was at a critical place on her path. He said that she had not demonstrated the proper amount of faith when she allowed herself to be persuaded by family and friends that the cancer must continue to be a source of fear. I was to let her know that she would be fine if she did not divert too much from the path which was being shown to her. She would live long enough to do her work, accomplish her growth and die peacefully when she had fulfilled her assignments.

Then a most remarkable thing occurred. LU CHOW PIN asked to speak with me. EKETAN acceded to this request. He suggested that acupuncture was in order at this time. I asked LU CHOW PIN to tell me what points to needle. He began to name the points in Chinese. I am not competent in locating acupuncture points by Chinese names, but I can recognize the names as Chinese. I asked LU CHOW PIN to tell me the points he wanted needled according to the western system of meridian name and point number. He did not know the points by meridian name and point number. I thought for a minute and asked if he would use Samantha's finger to indicate precisely where he wanted the needles placed. (I should mention that all of this dialogue was going through Samantha as she assumed her Oriental face and quiet English speaking voice with the unmistakable Oriental accent.)

Without much hesitation, Samantha's right index finger (attached to her hand, of course) pointed to Large Intestine 4, Triple Heater 8, Gallbladder 4 and Liver 8. LU CHOW PIN said, "You will place needles at these points—on both sides, of course."

I thought I would try to be helpful and explain the name and number system that we use to identify acupuncture points. LU CHOW PIN said that this information was of no interest to him. Later, Samantha denied any previous knowledge of acupuncture point names and locations.

Then, HAWKINS' wonderful British voice came through Samantha's throat. He told me that I was too serious. He said that he wished he could get out with me and have a drink or two. I asked if he could go home with me that evening after work. He said that he could. I asked, "If I drink champagne and you are with me, could you also enjoy it?" He said, "Jolly well would like that." I did go home after work and open a bottle of champagne. I was home alone that evening, so I sat with the champagne and talked to HAWKINS. That night he told me not to worry; he would always be with me to correct my course whenever I might need an adjustment. I just needed to stay open. There I was drinking champagne and talking to myself!

But let me return to the session with Samantha. EKETAN came back before the session was over. He told me that he had a special interest in my work because we had worked together in Egypt. We had been physicians working on the correction of brain disease that caused paralysis. I asked, "Disease?" He asked that I please forgive him; he did not understand all the nuances of the language; he meant "brain injury." He said that all I must do was to remain open.

I did not see Samantha and her friends again until March 8, 1989. She stated that the arm, shoulder and neck was more persistent. She had gone back on the fast track in business to some extent—not as much as before, but she had made no further moves toward developing a service/teaching career. I thought the pain to be an attention-getter. No structural problem came to my attention. Energy seemed focused and disorganized around the nipple of the left breast. The right breast seemed quiet and organized.

The guide who came forth at this session was CHAMAAS. (I always have them spell their names if they will.) CHAMAAS said that he needed help from me with the lower vibration levels, while he worked on the development of her higher development levels. He requested that I see her weekly for awhile. I agreed to do whatever CHAMAAS wanted/suggested, of course. I didn't know what I was doing, but he said I knew on a deeper level because I was doing precisely what he wanted me to do. I am not yet intellectually sure what I was doing in that session. I just thought "lower vibration" in my mind and let my hands do whatever they wanted to do.

Samantha returned on March 14. This time, the guide was JABOOM. He asked me if I had gotten his messages. I said that I didn't know. I added that I had felt closed this past week and I apologized. He told me not to expect perfection when working in an earthly body. I was doing fine.

Samantha was amnesic for both the March 9 and March 14 sessions. She had to accept my word that the pain existed to let her know that she was still not giving proper freedom to her femaleness. She must be a woman. She was having trouble letting go of the success and acclaim she had achieved as a business professional. (Actually, she was a vice president of a rather large architectural development firm.)

The next time I saw Samantha on March 23, she said she would not be able to come back to see me again because the insurance wouldn't pay any more. She would not lie down on the table, but it was a good session. She ventilated a lot of anger about this whole thing. We discussed her "spoiled child syndrome," her anger at being directed by spirit guides to do something that involved serious life change, risk and sacrifice—and she wanted this shoulder pain gone. Also, she wanted proof that the cancer had not come back. We discussed trust. I told her that if she wanted a mammogram, ultrasound, Trans Illumination and some blood tests I would order them. She should think about it for a week or so—she could go in and get the tests or not; it was her decision. I made it clear that whether or not she got the tests would reflect the level of her trust.

I next saw Samantha on April 14. She had done the tests and they were all negative for any suspicion of cancer. We talked about trust, her resistance to the unfolding of her path and so on. She had calmed down. The pressure from her family to continually search for cancer was immense. She had a hard time resisting. They couldn't believe that she could be cancer-free without having followed the doctors' recommendations. She also got cards from doctors that disclaimed responsibility for her being well since she hadn't complied with their recommendations. We got all of this conversation out of the way, then a vault hold, a little balancing, a Still Point and Samantha was once again in her altered state of consciousness. A deep voice came from her. It said, "Greetings, my son. I am BAKANANDA. I have taken charge for the time being. I shall instruct you. He then told me to use my energy to open the glands and ducts of the left breast, thorax, shoulder and neck. I tried to comply. BAKANANDA said I was doing it just right. I could feel the tissue response.

I then screwed up my courage and asked BAKANANDA if we could image away the fibrocystic breast disease. He said, "Certainly you can, but it is no concern to those on my plane. That Samantha works on fibrocystic tissue is irrelevant." I took this as a "yes." After Samantha came back to the present time and place, we practiced imaging together what her breast tissue would look like if it were normal. She agreed to spend perhaps 15 minutes a day on this work. I hoped that palpable improvement in the texture of her breast tissue would give her what she needed.

Samantha returned to see me on April 27. She went into her altered state almost as soon as she lay down on the table. Once again, BAKANANDA came through as the spiritual guide. He advised me that I should now tell Samantha why she was having so much trouble during the past few months. He told me that

Samantha had been a slave in Egypt. She had been freed from her enslavement by a group of rebels. She then came to power and enslaved the very people who had liberated her. Now, she was still carrying the burden of that guilt with her. In addition to her rejection of femininity—some of which was due to her enslavement as a female during this lifetime—she also had to let go of her guilt for turning upon her liberators before she could totally uproot the rest of her problem.

BAKANANDA then instructed me to energize her spleen and then to open her root chakra (energy center). I did this without difficulty. Things always seem to go easily when you are doing what you are told to do by a spirit guide. I let BAKANANDA know how easy it was for me to work when I am guided. He told me that it was a pleasure to work with me because I did not question what I was guided to do. I then asked him how I could know when a sense of being guided was authentic. He said that when it was true I would feel my solar plexus vibrate. If I was being misled, either by myself or by an inferior spirit, I would feel nothing in my solar plexus. So now I'm trying to be aware of my solar plexus when an idea comes to mind.

I then asked BAKANANDA if I could gain some further understanding from him about my life. He said he would help in any way that he could. I explained that I felt that the teaching of high purpose intentioned touch was a way of diffusing anger and violence. He told me that he knew about that and what we were doing. He stated that it is a part of what needs to be done. I asked him how we could finance the continuation of our work. BAKANANDA said that finance was of no concern on the higher vibratory levels. I told him that we exist on this level, so money has to be a concern to us. Strangely, he responded that he had forgotten that we have a M-O-N-E-T-A-R-Y (he spelled the word) system to deal with. It was of no spiritual significance and was just one of those ridiculous things the beings on a lower vibrational plane create in order to make life more difficult and complex. He said that they would help as they could, but since it was a system created by incarnate beings, it required that it be dealt with primarily on the incarnate level. That answered my question quite clearly: He said that we had to keep on working in the trenches. It may also explain why so many good, spiritually focused projects go bankrupt.

I thanked BAKANANDA for the information he had imparted. I asked if there was anything else he wished to tell me or to have me do before we ended this session. He reminded me to gently help Samantha understand the guilt she was carrying for enslaving her liberators back in Egypt.

I gently tried to tell Samantha about the Egyptian experience after she awakened. She could recall no part of our session. She had to take my word for it if she were to believe it, accept it and act on it. This required real trust. It didn't help that her left shoulder was still a little painful. The pain suggested to me, however, that her level of trust was not quite what it should be. We discussed this mild deficit in her trust and Samantha agreed to work on it. We then agreed that we would work together about once a month for as long as we felt it to be beneficial.

I next saw Samantha on May 31. She still had some shoulder pain and was mildly upset about it. She wanted some tests done to get to the bottom of this pain. I told her that we could get the tests but that I thought we were already at the bottom of the pain and she just didn't want to see it. (We remained friends even though I said this to her.) I did order an arthritis profile blood test as well as a Chem Screen (multifaceted screening blood test). Two days later, both came back as normal.

But back to the May 31 session. After we drew the blood, Samantha settled down. She had gotten what she needed; now she was ready to work again. She lay on the table and I began balancing her craniosacral system from the vault. She went into a very nice relaxed state. Very suddenly, her craniosacral rhythm stopped. The Significance Detector indicated that something was happening.

I asked who was there. A beautiful, loving, feminine voice responded, "It is I, my son, SOUL OF EGYPT. I was surrounded by the most loving, quieting, safe and wonderful atmosphere I had ever experienced. I asked what SOUL OF EGYPT would have me do. This wonderful voice said, "Touch and listen."

Remember the first time you saw the boy or girl of your dreams and fell madly in love? I felt like that. I was tingling from head to toe. I was definitely in love with SOUL OF EGYPT. I asked her for a name by which I could address her. She said SOUL OF EGYPT was all that she wished to tell me.

She then went on to say that she was the soul of Samantha when she was a slave to the pharaoh. She described herself as very beautiful with dark eyes, long black hair, beautiful olive tanned skin and so on. In return for some political favors, her father had given her to the pharaoh when she was only 15 years of age. Soon, the pharaoh began abusing her sexually. SOUL OF EGYPT described how the pharaoh drank too much wine every night. This prevented him from gaining an erection. In response to his own sexual impotency, he would become angry. He would then insert into her vagina a wand made of silver and inset with precious stones and ravage her in this way. Each time he did this he became more violent until he finally penetrated into her pelvic cavity and she died after a few days of hemorrhage and infection. I now had to release this Energy Cyst and its attendant emotion. The release went well. I simply put one hand over the vaginal area (Samantha was wearing street clothes) and the other hand over the left and middle anterior pelvic wall. The release came very easily and was very powerful as an energy vector coming back out of the vagina. I imagined that I could feel the pharaoh's rage and frustration as it exited her body. Maybe I did feel it; I'm not sure of these things any more.

SOUL OF EGYPT then thanked me for being so helpful. She bade me farewell and I could feel the wonderful vibrations gently and slowly leave the room.

There I sat, with my hands on Samantha's pelvis, almost totally in shock. I went back up to Samantha's head, collected my wits and brought her back to the present.

As usual, she remembered nothing. As I described SOUL OF EGYPT, Samantha's eyes shined like I have never seen them shine before. She softened and seemed to suddenly trust. I told her about her experiences with the pharaoh, about her death. I tried to help her accept what had happened. I described how the pharaoh's energies were released from her body. She told me that this felt like another part of the reason she was denying her femininity in this lifetime.

It was a good session with a good closure. When I think about SOUL OF EGYPT, I still feel totally in awe and somewhat like a smitten teenager.

I called Samantha in a couple of days to let her know that her laboratory results were normal. For the first time, she seemed disinterested. She said that she knew they were normal and would look forward to seeing me in three or four weeks.

My last visit with Samantha before writing this account of our experiences together occurred on June 28, 1989. She was in good spirits on that date. She no longer seemed worried about the presence of cancer in her body. We chatted a little while as I began working with her craniosacral system. The urgency to go into deep trance seemed less dominant. After a few minutes, I asked whether there was anyone who would like to speak with us today. Within a minute or so after my inquiry, Samantha was deep into her altered state of consciousness. A gentle feminine voice came from Samantha. The voice informed us that her name was EUJUTA and told us that SOUL OF EGYPT sends love. EUJUTA then told me that I must continue to work with Samantha until her heart chakra (energy center) remains open and flowing. She told me, in response to my questions, that about once a month should be fine.

Next, EUJUTA wanted to give us some information regarding physical sex and spiritual love. She stated that physical sex with love in the proper setting promoted spiritual connection between the participants. This spiritual union promoted unconditional love and thus spiritual evolution. Physical sex without high spiritual meaning was for lust. Lust obstructs the path towards spiritual advancement.

Monogamy on the physical plane is a human creation of little spiritual importance except that it may get in the way of the union of several spirits who may be ready to connect. However, we must know that physical sex is not required for spiritual connection. It does, however, facilitate that spiritual connection when the physical sex is done with good intent rather than for reasons of lust.

With these comments, EUJUTA departed the session. The heart chakra (energy center) was open. Since she is a single woman, I expect that EUJUTA's comments about spiritual love and its relationship to physical sex were meant to clarify some confusion in Samantha's mind. (We'll see what the future holds.)

Before closing this chapter, I want to share one more experience with you that might further clarify the question of channeling as it has presented itself to me. This subject is a 41-year-old male named Gary who first came to us during the summer of 1988. I did not see him during that time. He was treated by one of the other osteopathic physicians here at The Institute.

The man returned for a week of treatments in November 1988. During this time, I did one session with him. During this session, he re-experienced and went through the SomatoEmotional Release of his tonsillectomy and then his birth trauma.

In June of 1989, Gary returned for another week of treatments. This time, I had four sessions with him. During the first session, I worked toward the release of a chronic left arm and shoulder pain syndrome. During the second session, his voice changed and he spoke with me as an individual who called himself IM. IM told me that there was a group of scientists who were near to perfecting a "time suspension" machine. This machine was capable of suspending the passage of time for a given individual. Gary was to see that this was used for good and not for wrongful purposes. Gary was to discuss this with Mr. Gorbachev of the Soviet Union. Later, at the end of this session, I determined that Gary and Gorbachev with some others were, indeed, to have a meeting in the late summer of 1989. (Gary had sketchy memory for the content of this session when he returned to full consciousness.)

I had two more sessions with Gary during that week. We did some rather routine upper thoracic and cervical structural work. IM returned during both of these sessions with information for me. He stated that he was the messenger. He did not understand the meaning but I was to think about this, as it would ultimately be very important in my own work. IM then proceeded to describe a cylinder made of transparent lucite material mounted in a gyro-type machine. Within this cylinder, he described what I interpreted to be the double helix of DNA. IM didn't know what it was; he said that he could only describe it. He also told me that it had to do with the work we were doing against the spread of violence. He could tell me no more. That was it.

These are some of the more outstanding experiences that I have had while working with patients. Dismissal of these experiences as nonconscious parts making their presence known—or perhaps as multiple personality disorder manifestations or even as psychotic episodes can be made. (And you can make a case for either the patient or myself being the psychotic one.) But if you are there, it isn't quite so easy to write them off as non-spiritual experiences. In the previous chapter (which describes my personal experiences), it is made clear that I was a firm skeptic some years ago. Now, I'm quite open and leaning toward the idea that there are spirit guides who offer a lot of very good wisdom to those of us who will accept it.

I'm sure that I have accepted a lot of wise advice for many years, even while I thought I was a skeptic.

The events I have described did occur. Most often, there was a preceptor witness in the room with us. So there is verification of the events described. There were several other such experiences. Those I have described here are exemplary.

I can't end this chapter without sharing one more experience that I had with another female patient. Her guide, SARAH, was communicating with me freely and offering advice and wisdom throughout the session. Finally, I asked SARAH if there was anything else she would like me to do before ending the session. SARAH was quiet for a minute and then said, "No, I think we've done what was necessary." I thanked her and asked if it was okay if I "popped" the seventh cervical vertebra on the right side. SARAH said, "Go ahead if you think you should, but wait a minute until I get out of here." I waited a few seconds. I'm sure I felt an energy change. Then I used a direct thrust on C7. The patient awakened within seconds after the "POP." She exclaimed, "You've popped my neck."

CHANNELING POSTSCRIPT

After proofreading this manuscript, I had occasion to have another visit with Samantha. I had a preceptor named Harvey with me. To the best of our recollection, the dialogue content is paraphrased below. Neither of us will ever forget this experience.

Samantha came into the session in a very positive mood. She stated that she was still working as a business professional and that she was participating as one of the sponsors in an "energy healing" seminar that weekend. She was elated about this opportunity.

She had only one concern about her body at the time of this visit. There was a small but palpable lump in her left axilla. She pointed it out to me, and it was definitely there. It was about the size of a pea. I think that I was more concerned than she was because I put on my traditional physician's hat immediately and started to worry that this lump might be a metastatic tumor spread from her left breast which was the site of her original (as far as we know) malignancy.

I tuned into her craniosacral rhythm with a vault hold. Harvey sat near her head as a silent observer. She relaxed easily. Within just a few minutes she was deep in a relaxed trance-like state. I asked very gently and quietly if there was anyone there who would advise and help us during the session that day. Her face sort of screwed up around her mouth and her lips pursed. A rather deep voice said, "There are two." I misunderstood and thought that I was encountering an entity named "Too" or Tuo." I enquired about the spelling. The voice from Samantha became a little impatient sounding and said, "There are two today." There was a little interchange about "two," "too" and "tuo," an apology on my part and then the voice from Samantha introduced itself as JAMOOZE. I commented on the beauty and uniqueness of the names of the guides I had encountered during my work with Samantha. JAMOOZE explained that the names were created by those on his plane for our benefit as we worked because we seemed to need names. On his plane they had no use for names. This is why, sometimes, they are slow to respond when we ask for a given entity by name. They are not accustomed to the use of names as we on earth know and use them. JAMOOZE said that all entities on higher planes know one another by vibration. He then said that HAWKINS sent me his love.

JAMOOZE informed me that all was going well with Samantha. He said that the "hardness" in the breast where the surgical biopsy had been done was breaking up and dissolving. I asked about the lump that Samantha had pointed out to me. He said, "You mean in the pit arm?" I didn't understand "pit arm." He repeated, "pit arm," a little impatiently, and I finally realized what he meant. I said, "Oh, you mean the armpit?" He just mumbled something about "pit arm, arm pit, what is the difference?"

JAMOOZE directed me to open the channel between the root and the crown chakras through the vertical core of her body. He then instructed me to use Harvey's hands in addition to my own. He said that Harvey was not there by accident; his connection was desired. Harvey was to open the lower body core with one hand and do the spleen with the other. I used one hand on the crown chakra, and then at JAMOOZE's instruction, I placed one finger on the lump in Samantha's "pit arm." JAMOOZE told us to connect the upper and lower body by opening the core. At the same time, Harvey was to energize the spleen while I dissolved the lump. In a matter of a few minutes, it all worked just as JAMOOZE said it would.

Samantha's face went all soft and radiant. You could feel the love in the air. You could almost cut it with a knife, it was so prominent. A beautiful voice issued forth from Samantha's new face. The voice said, "I am ILNA. I come to bring love and gentleness to this healing." ILNA then told me that Samantha was doing extremely well. All I had to do from now on was to be sure the heart chakra remained open. She said, "It is necessary that the heart chakra remain open so that love can flow freely in and out. There can be no disease when the heart chakra is open and love flows freely." ILNA then made a flat statement that allowed for no discussion or argument. She said, "There is no disease without conflict." I repeated it three or four times to be sure there were no questions about what I understood. ILNA repeated again after each of my responses, "Yes, my son. It is true. There is no disease without conflict." I finally understood that, without exception, there is no question about the broad application of this statement.

Then, a statement came from ILNA that took me totally by surprise. She said, "Print twice as many copies of your book as you think you should. It will be very much in demand." I asked her what book she meant. She said the book I was just finishing. Then, she told me that they were all pleased that I had followed their suggestions. I asked what suggestion that was. ILNA said that about a year before they told me to begin writing this book. I had objected a little, but when they gave me the message to sit down and start writing, I did, and they were pleased.

I then said that as long as we were on the topic of the book, perhaps she could help with a question that we were discussing. This question involved the possible loss of credibility I might suffer by putting into print the rather detailed descriptions of some of the rather incredible experiences in which I have been privileged to be a participant. We were just beginning to discuss the possibility of editing out some of the more far-out descriptions for fear of losing some of our developing support.

ILNA said simply, "Do not edit; stand on your feet; put your head up and tell the truth." There wasn't much room for doubt about her statement. Everything I have written is the truth to the best of my ability to remember and know; it should not be edited. ILNA then went on to say that those who were close to me who advised editing did not know that the time was right nor understand the importance of the message. Some would have difficulty with what I have presented. She hoped that they would be challenged to evolve and grow to new levels of advancement, but if not, that was each one's individual choice. ILNA then said, "Be at peace, my son. We are pleased." She left.

Samantha slowly came back to the here and now. I asked her to find the lump in her left armpit (or was it pit arm?). She couldn't find it and was very pleased.

I asked her if she knew I had just finished the pre-galley manuscript of a new book. She said, "No." Then she thought for a minute and said maybe she had heard something about me beginning a new book about a year before, but she wasn't sure.

So, my friends, the manuscript for the book you hold in your hands remains uncut. I have complete trust.

AFTERWORD

As the move toward balance and integration continues, events present at a
dizzying pace. Each time I proofed the first edition of this book, I was concerned
about the need to rewrite one section or another as it became dated or obsolete by
more recent happenings. (That trend continued with this edition.) If I were to do
that, I would rewrite ad infinitum and never publish: at some point in linear time,
a line must be drawn. I drew it in the last edition and included in the "Afterword"
some events about which I wanted to let the reader know.

Two of the most exciting include:

1. The successful documentation of the movement of the intracranial membranes of both embalmed and fresh, non-embalmed human cadavers when small
external forces were employed.

2. The successful recording of the change of electrically active phenomena
occurring during hands-on treatment of patients—not only by me but by another
physician with craniosacral orientation.

The membrane movement was recorded in two different ways during two separate investigatory efforts. In the first, Dimetrios Kostopoulous, P.T., recorded embalmed cadaveric falx cerebri movement in response to controlled frontal bone
traction using instruments which measured piezoelectrical current changes in the
falx cerebri membrane in response to tension changes.

Next, I had the opportunity to participate with physical therapist Cynthia
Rowe, physicist Neil Mohon and forensic photographer Michael J. Mahoney in an
attempt to palpate, observe and photographically document intracranial dura mater
movement and/or tension changes in a fresh, unembalmed cadaveric specimen.
The total brain was removed through a single two-inch-square opening made in
the right parietal bone. Such an opening was used in order to minimize the weak-
ening effect on the osseous integrity and strength of the skull. It did not cross a
sutural line. Neil applied measured forces to the outside of the body and placed
markers on the falx cerebelli. Michael recorded on film the movement of the dot-
markered dural structure in response to externally applied forces. Cynthia and i
both felt membrane tensions change as external forces were applied to the sacrum
and frontal bone as well as in response to the temporal ear pull technique. This was
an exciting beginning!

Later, one Saturday afternoon in January 1990, Neil (the same physicist) and
I, along with osteopaths Dick MacDonald and Bill Stager, got together to begin to
look for signs of energy transference between therapist/facilitator and patient/cli-
ent. We were able to clearly see the energy that occurred during treatment. This
energy exhibited electrical characteristics measurable in ohms. We saw the energy
readings change on the ohmmeter in synchronization and also in positive correlation to onset of treatment, encountering patient/client tissue resistance, tissue re-

lease and end of treatment as reported by the therapist/facilitator. We saw this same energy unimpaired by a series of materials imposed in the circuit established between therapist/facilitator and patient/client. The materials we tested included wood, styrofoam, rubber, aluminum, ultraviolet filter and a variety of fabrics.

And so it goes. Time and events race forward. It seems as though the master plan is saying it is time to integrate and balance the hard knowledge of science with the intuitive knowing of healing.

Godspeed,

John E. Upledger

John E. Upledger, D.O., O.M.M.

FACILITATED SEGMENTS
Reprinted from *CranioSacral Therapy Volume II, Beyond the Dura, pages 214 – 216*

This concept is relevant to neuromusculoskeletal as well as psychoemotional problems. Usually, the word "facilitated" has a positive connotation, implying that some process is made easier or more efficient. In the case of the "facilitated segment," however, it means that the stimulus threshold i.e., the resistance to the conduction of an electrical impulse in a particular spinal cord segment, has been reduced. This means that the facilitated segment of the spinal cord is highly excitable and that a smaller stimulus will trigger impulse firing in the segment.

This hypersensitivity may be detrimental to the body as a whole, depending on the tissue involved—for example, if the segment which innervates the stomach becomes facilitated, the stomach becomes hypersensitive. Therefore, mildly irritating food substances may cause disproportionately large pains and/or stomach dysfunctions. The person who has this problem may be said to have a nervous stomach or to possess food allergies or intolerances. If the situation continues, gastritis or ulceration may follow.

The concept of the facilitated segment originated in work done by Dr. I.M. Korr and his associates, beginning in the 1940s at the Kirksville College of Osteopathy and Surgery. The word "segment" means one of the parts into which something separates or divides. In the phrase "facilitated segment," the word can be somewhat misleading. It suggests that the spinal cord is naturally divided into pieces or segments. To some extent this is true, but we must keep in mind that both functionally and structurally the spinal cord is a longitudinal structure. It connects the brain with the nerve roots, which branch out to form the peripheral nervous system. The spinal cord can be analogized to a freeway and the spinal nerve roots to on ramps and off ramps. Although the spinal cord is a continuous structure, the nerve roots do branch off at regular intervals and can thus be viewed as delimiting "segments" of the spinal cord.

A spinal segment, in this sense, can be defined as a level of the spinal cord at which two dorsal nerve roots (sensory) enter and two ventral nerve roots (motor) exit. In a facilitated segment these roots are overly sensitive or hair triggered, as explained above. The hyperactive ventral motor root from the segment passes through the intervertebral foramen and joins the sympathetic nerve chain, which thereby comes under constant bombardment. This in turn keeps the sympathetic nervous system in a state of chronic overactivity, ultimately resulting in damage to the target organs and the patient's health. If the "trophic nerve function" hypothesis is true, this process may also result in protein deprivation in the target organs.

A facilitated segment produces a palpable change in tissue texture. The local paravertebral muscles and connective tissues develop a "shoddy" feel, and joints in the area are less mobile. The tissues are tender to the touch and often painfully irritable. I believe the that term "fibrositis" can be applied to the connective tissues in this situation. Sympathetic system dysfunction at the level of the facilitated segment also produces changes in skin texture, sweat gland activity and capillary supply to the skin.

Dr. Korr compares the facilitated segment to a "neuronal lens." By this he means that it seems to gather nerve impulses. It does not pass on its sensory input; rather, it accumulates and hoards not only those stimuli which come into it directly but also those which are attempting to pass through to other segments. Experimental electromyographic work done by Dr. Korr and his associates has demonstrated that increased stimulus of the nervous system almost everywhere will result in increased electrical activity of the muscle services by nerve roots derived from a facilitated segment.

Facilitated segments seem to occur at areas of focus for postural stress, sites of trauma and segmental levels related to visceral problems. Once established, a facilitated segment can continue for years, even ultimately contributing to death. A facilitated segment at T4 may cause decreased vitality of the heart, leading to blockage of coronary arteries and myocardial infarction. A facilitated segment tends to perpetuate itself. That is, the hyperactivity of the motor root causes the related sympathetic ganglion to become hyperactive, leading to dysfunction and deterioration of the target organs. A variety of sensory stimuli related to the dysfunction are sent back to the spinal segment, further increasing its level of facilitation and so on. Different types of problems are associated with facilitated segment at specific levels e.g. T9/10 (gallbladder), T12/L1 (kidney), L5 (urogenital), etc. Once a segment becomes facilitated, all associated target structures (connective tissue, muscle, bone, blood vessels, skin, sweat glands and internal organs) will be adversely affected.

Therapeutically, any approach which interrupts the self-perpetuating activity of the facilitated segment will be helpful. The sensory input to the segment must be reduced. Effective approaches, therefore, include those which: (1) relax the muscles (massage, soft tissue manipulation); (2) mobilize the area and thus reduce stasis and edema (structural manipulative therapy); (3) reduce postural stress (Rolfing, Alexander Technique); (4) reduce the number of signals from higher centers of the central nervous system (relaxation techniques, biofeedback, hypnotherapy, tranquilizers); (5) combine those effects (osteopathic manipulative treatment). CranioSacral Therapy is also very helpful in that it reduces autonomic tonus (sympathetic activity), reduces general stress and anxiety, helps endocrine function, assists in postural balancing and improves fluid exchange.

CHAKRAS
Reprinted from *CranioSacral Therapy Volume II, Beyond the Dura,*
Glossary of Terms and Concepts

These [*chakras*] have been conceptualized by yogis in India since ancient times as centers of the ethereal body (energy body which engulfs the physical body) which take in vitality (*prahna*) from the surrounding atmosphere in order to energize the individual. In general, chakras are best palpated just off the physical body of the patient, although touching is permissible. They can range from 3 – 15 cm in diameter. In my perception, the first six of the chakras below are associated with energy fields which spin clockwise. There are seven chakras which are palpable to me:

The root *chakram* is related to sexuality and reproduction and is said to be the seat of the *"Kundalini"* (fiery serpent). Kundalini is thought to be an energy derived from the sun, stored at the base of the spine and, when liberated, rushes up the spinal canal to the brain, activating all the chakras as it passes them. I have treated a few advanced yogis who said that CranioSacral Therapy enhanced and made easier the ascent of their Kundalini. The root chakra is palpable in the supine patient with one hand placed under the sacrum and the other, very lightly, on the lower abdomen just above the symphysis pubis. I have found this chakram to be active most frequently in women who have an unsatisfactory sexual life, especially those who trade sex for material support with no feelings of love. Opening this chakram and the heart chakram simultaneously will frequently improve and integrate the sexual and love relationships.

The navel chakram is related to sensitivity, feelings and emotions, as well as the function of the liver, kidneys, intestines, digestion and solar plexus. It is best palpated with one hand under the upper and middle lumbar spine and the other just below the navel, barely touching the body.

The spleen chakram is related to the assimilation of energy and its distribution to the other parts of the body; it is similar to the concept found in the acupuncture theory of the spleen as the refiner and distributor of *chi* to the other organs. This chakram is best palpated with one hand holding the thoracolumbar junction and the other placed very lightly over the epigastrium. Improving the function of this chakram will often improve immunity, resistance and general activity levels.

The heart chakram is best palpated with one hand under the mid-thoracic spine and the other hand just touching the mid-sternal area. In my experience, this chakram is frequently dysfunctional in those who have been hurt as children by someone in whom they had great trust. Now they are afraid to love for fear of being hurt again. The heart and root chakras are frequently dysfunctional together in women whose marriages involve sex without love.

The throat chakram is best palpated with one hand cradling the back of the neck and the other covering the thyroid cartilage, with a thumb and finger on the two upper lateral extremities of the cartilage. Frequently the chakram is felt as two separate energy centers, each spinning clockwise on the two sides of the throat; I believe this is normal. This chakram has to do with communication with other people and the ability to express one's feelings verbally.

Index